CONTENTS

Acknowledgements

We are extremely grateful to Deborah Colson, who is not only an excellent nutritionist but also an expert in GL and who has done sterling work calculating the GL scores of all the recipes. We would also like to thank everyone at Piatkus, especially Jo Brooks, for bringing this book to completion.

I (Fiona) would also like to thank the entire Holford and Associates team, for their advice and taste testing; the Harbour crowd, particularly my sister Sophie, for endless support and cups of mint tea; and my incredibly tolerant parents, who allowed me to take over their kitchen for the past year. Last but most definitely not least I would like to thank Nick, for being an all-round splendid chap. And I (Patrick) would like to thank Charlotte, my super-efficient PA, and Gaby, my wonderful wife, for their support and encouragement.

patrick HOLFORD
and Fiona McDonald Joyce

THE
LOW-GL
DIET
COOKBOOK

piatkus

PIATKUS

First published in Great Britain in 2005 by Piatkus Books as
The Holford Low-GL Diet Cookbook
Reprinted 2006, 2007, 2009, 2012
This edition published as *The Low-GL Diet Cookbook* in 2010

13 15 17 19 20 18 16 14

A CIP catalogue record for this book
is available from the British Library.

ISBN 978-0-7499-2642-7

Designed by Smith & Gilmour, London
Edited by Barbara Kiser
Proofread by Libby Willis
Index compiled by Lisa Footitt

Photography by Liberty Silver, except pages 8, 40, 49 and 65

Printed and bound by C&C Offset

Piatkus
An imprint of
Little, Brown Book Group
Carmelite House
50 Victoria Embankment
London EC4Y 0DZ

An Hachette UK Company
www.hachette.co.uk

www.improvementzone.co.uk

INTRODUCTION

Ever felt that food itself – that simple, pleasurable thing – has become a minefield? We're constantly bombarded with statistics on how obesity is rocketing in the West, and articles that reveal many 'school meals' to be thinly disguised junk food. So healthy eating is very much on our minds, and many of us are eager to lose weight – on doctors' orders, or simply to feel better about ourselves.

As a result, an avalanche of diet books has hit the shelves. They promise the world but deliver complicated, unsatisfying, expensive and sometimes downright dangerous information. If you've sampled any of them, you'll be fed up with jumping from one 'miracle' diet to the next. But now you've found a place to linger. This book is a gimmick-free zone with not an empty promise in sight. The information in its pages is backed by more than two decades' worth of research by the Institute for Optimum Nutrition, or ION, which I founded in 1984. Over that time we have found a way to lose weight and feel great for life. The result is the Holford Diet.

We have worked out that if you want to shed extra pounds and feel fantastic, all you need to do is follow two simple rules:

Eat a 'low-GL' diet (more on that in a moment)
Eat carbohydrate with protein

This book is designed to make following these rules painless by providing recipes that balance everything out for you. As you'll see – and know, if you've tried the recipes in my book *The Low-GL Diet Bible* – this is food with zing. It's fresh, tasty, satisfying, simple to source and prepare, and rich in the kind of nutrients you need to cope with life 21st-century style.

To be honest, I'm no natural-born cook. Unlike Fiona, my co-author, who lives and breathes cookery and is forever trying out new dishes on me and my team, I give up easily if a recipe is too complicated or takes too long. But that's not what this cookbook is about. I can vouch for the fact that not only do the finished products taste completely delicious and help you look and feel good, they're also dead easy to follow. If I can make them, you can make them! And they'll work in any context, from Sunday breakfast and teenage feasts to formal dinners.

Finding the balance

But this book delivers something much more powerful than over 150 recipes, however mouthwatering.

Do you remember when you learned to ride a bike? The actual moment when you 'got' balance, after endlessly falling to the left or right? That's exactly what *The Low-GL Diet Cookbook* is about – learning a new distinction that we call 'GL balance'. GL, or Glycemic Load, is a better way of gauging the effect of foods on your blood sugar levels (and thus your energy, wellbeing and weight) than the now-familiar Glycemic Index (GI). And it's very easy to get to grips with. You will not only learn which foods have a low GL, you'll also develop a new sensitivity to your own blood sugar levels.

So instead of reaching unconsciously for a chocolate bar or cup of coffee when your energy levels dip, you'll find yourself aware that it's time to eat one of the many low-GL snacks offered in this book. You won't be 'dying of hunger' – you'll just need to eat something! And because you'll find the food boosting your energy for much longer, and much more evenly, than sweets and stimulants ever can, you'll find yourself sticking with this way of eating. It's only this kind of permanent, internal learning that leads to a permanent change in your weight, your health and your energy.

With so many other diets out there making miraculous claims but failing to deliver, you might be sceptical at this point – which is perfectly understandable. The difference with this approach is that it has been tried and tested over decades. Since I founded ION, more than 100,000 volunteers have put my ideas into practice, and the success stories have been legion.

Ellen's story is one of them. She was a typical stressed-out 30-year-old working woman in London, and GMTV challenged me to give her a health transformation in 10 days. What needed transforming? Ellen used to wake up tired, without any energy, in desperate need of a coffee to kickstart her enthusiasm for the day. Her skin was dry and flaky. She was constantly getting colds and was too tired to exercise, despite having previously loved running. She felt low a lot of the time and experienced frequent mood swings. To try to stop gaining any more weight, she'd avoid breakfast – except for a coffee – and would snack off fruit, while often succumbing to other, less healthful treats. She'd usually end her day by eating fast food or pre-prepared dishes from the supermarket, washed down with wine to help her get to sleep.

She was not delighted when I told her to eat more food! To have breakfast every day, a substantial lunch and dinner, and two snacks, Holford Diet style. I also recommended a few supplements.

Ten days later, Ellen was a different woman. Here's what she said:

> **I'm waking up feeling refreshed and happy. I really enjoy my breakfast, which I didn't think I would do. I've lost 4lb despite eating more. I have the energy to go running and am now running at the weekend. My concentration is vastly improved at work. I'm more alert and on the ball. I've also noticed a definite improvement in my skin. The flakiness and dryness have gone, not only on my face but on my body as well. My mood is more even. I have no sniffles and snuffles. I'm coping better with stress.**

It really is that easy. How you feel and how you look are the direct consequence of the action you take today. If you feel hopelessly embedded in 'bad' eating habits that you know are hampering your full enjoyment of life, what you'll find in this book is a simple plan for taking action. It doesn't involve rigid discipline, hunger pangs, expensive foods or boredom. We've worked it out to be a completely easy and enjoyable transition to a new life, and within two weeks it will become a habit – a positive, life-changing one that has you waking up full of energy and free of cravings.

Wishing you happy cooking and the best of health!

Patrick Holford

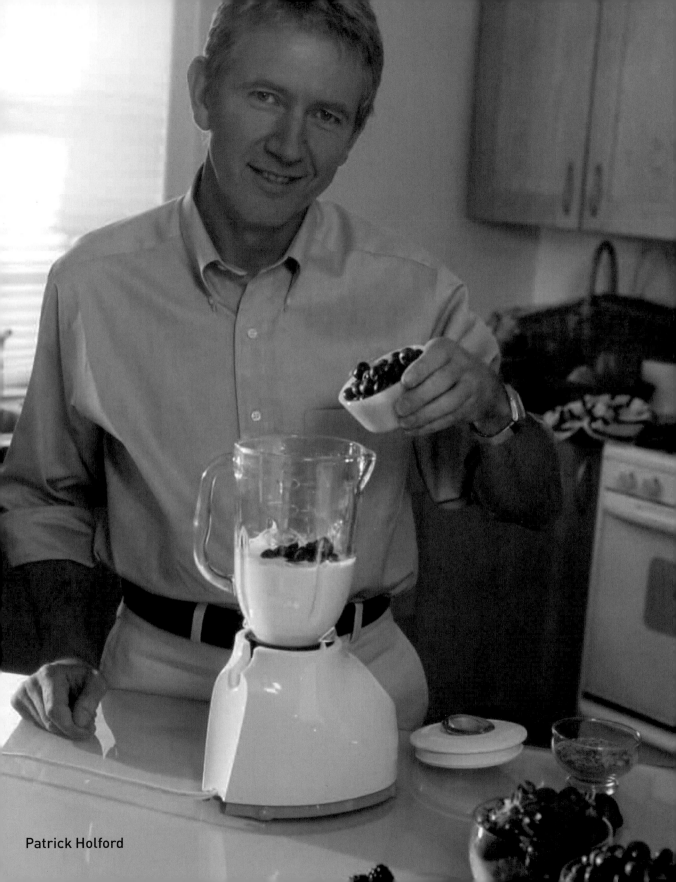

Patrick Holford

HOW TO USE THIS BOOK

PART ONE gives you the key principles of the Holford Diet in a nutshell. We also recommend that you read *The Low-GL Diet Bible* for more detailed information, including the right supplements to take when you want to lose weight, and the kind of exercise that will best help you.

PART TWO gives you menu plans and more than 150 mouthwatering recipes to choose from. All you have to do each day is choose recipes and drinks that add up to no more than 45 ⓖⓛ if you want to lose weight, or 65 ⓖⓛ if you want to maintain weight.

PART 1:
SIX STEPS TO SUPERHEALTH

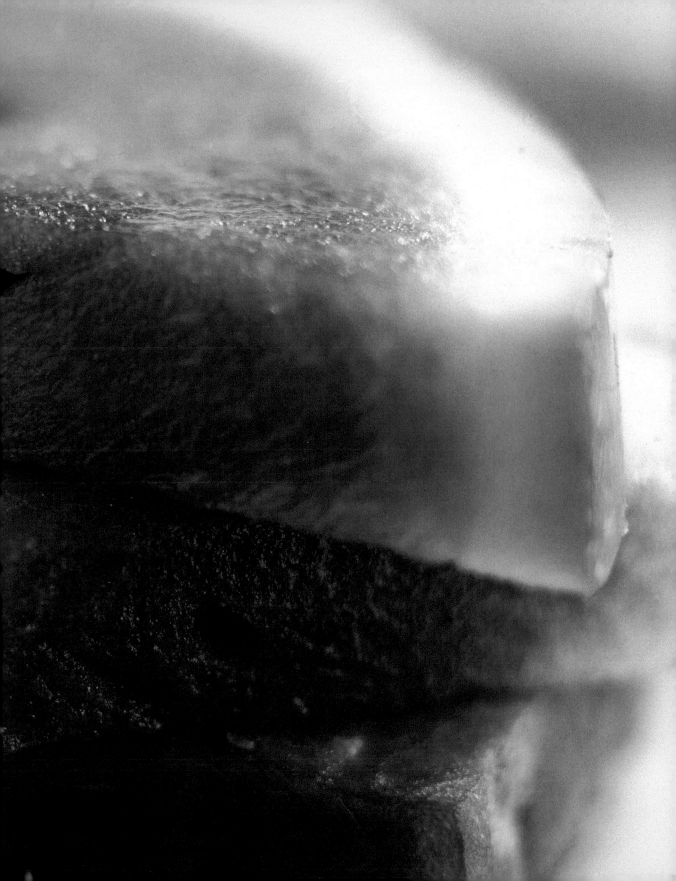

Eat the right GLs for your needs

The GL, or Glycemic Load, of a food or meal tells you exactly what it's going to do to your blood sugar – and hence, to your weight and energy levels. By eating no more than 40 Ⓖ a day, you keep it all in balance and lose weight. And when you've reached the maintenance phase, you can up your Ⓖ to 55 a day. Extra Ⓖ from drinks and puddings (see opposite) will up these totals to 45 and 65.

Go for protein/carb combinations

Holford Diet recipes mix protein with low-GL carbohydrates. Combining the two is another way of stabilizing blood sugar, staving off hunger and cutting out food cravings.

Graze, don't gorge

By spreading Ⓖ throughout the day – with 10 for breakfast, lunch and dinner and two 5 Ⓖ snacks – you'll avoid energy dips and keep hunger at bay.

Choose good fats, avoid bad ones

Your body needs – and craves – fat. When you eat enough of the essential omega-3 and omega-6 fats, you stop craving harmful processed, damaged and saturated fats.

Opt for the best drinks and puddings

You'll have extra ⓖⓑ for drinks and puddings – 5 or 10, depending on whether you're on the weight loss or maintenance plan.

Avoid allergy foods

Allergies to wheat and dairy products are very common, and a big source of weight gain. If this is the case for you, Holford Diet recipes will offer a huge range of options.

EAT THE RIGHT GLS FOR YOUR NEEDS

GL or Glycemic Load – the backbone of the Holford Diet – is a tool that tells you exactly what a particular food or meal will do to your blood sugar. This deceptively simple piece of information is dietary gold dust, because your blood sugar levels are intimately connected with hunger, and so with how we eat.

If you need to lose weight, you'll be eating 40 Ⓖⓛ a day on the Holford Diet (with an extra 5 Ⓖⓛ for drinks or puddings), and once you've reached the maintenance stage, you'll be eating a basic 55 Ⓖⓛ a day (plus an extra 10 Ⓖⓛ for drinks and desserts). But to fully understand GL, we need to take a quick look at the process of how your body converts carbohydrates into blood sugar.

Carbs and blood sugar: the cycle explained

Carbohydrates are the sugars and starches found in, well, sugar – and in cereal grains, fruits, beans and vegetables. When you haven't eaten any for a while, your blood sugar – the body's main fuel – dips and you become hungry. Then you eat a carbohydrate and your blood sugar levels rise. That's good – unless you're eating refined carbohydrates such as sugar. These cause your blood sugar levels to shoot up. Unable to use it all, your body dumps the excess as fat. Your blood sugar levels then crash . . . so you're left hungry again, lethargic, and craving more food as well as stimulants such as coffee or cigarettes. Eventually a vicious cycle of cravings, exhaustion and accumulating fat can set in.

It's clear that the food we eat needs to keep our blood sugar levels balanced. Take a look at the charts below, which compare how different foods affect our blood sugar levels.

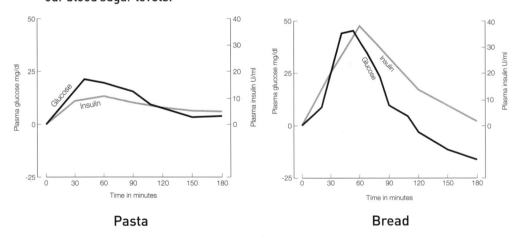

Pasta

Bread

So, how do you know which carbohydrate foods keep your blood sugar on an even keel – and which ones don't? (Proteins, as we'll see later, have a negligible effect on blood sugar.) The answer is GL.

All about GL

GL is a much more accurate and practical tool than the well-known GI, or Glycemic Index. In essence, GL builds on GI – so let's take a look at that.

GI is a way of scoring how fast the carbohydrate within a food raises your blood sugar compared with pure glucose. Carbohydrates in foods differ a lot in this respect. Apples, for instance, contain the carbohydrate fructose, which is slow-releasing. Sucrose, or table sugar, is fast-releasing. (Think two-star and four-star fuel.) The fastest-releasing of all is glucose, which is identical to blood sugar – five-star rocket fuel, in fact! Glucose, the benchmark, has a GI of 100. Fructose has a GI of 39. In practice, that means you'd have to eat roughly three times as much fructose to achieve the same increase in blood sugar as that triggered by pure glucose.

So GI tells you about the quality of carbohydrate in a food – that is, whether it is slow or fast-releasing. This is very useful, but only up to a point. For GI tells us nothing about how much carbohydrate a food contains – quantity, in short. (This is known as 'available carbohydrate', or net carbs minus indigestible fibre.) And that makes GI-based diets potentially misleading.

Why GL is better

GL goes one better than GI by factoring in both the quantity of carbs in a food, and its quality. To make clear why this is important, let's look at watermelon. Its GI is pretty high, at about 72. So the sugar in watermelon is fast-releasing. But when we look at it more closely, a very different picture emerges. Take a great big 120g slice of watermelon, and out of all that, only 6g counts as available carbohydrate! As its name implies, most of this fabulous fruit is actually water.

You work out GL using a simple equation, as shown in this box.

How to work out the GL of a food

Take the GI score   **multiplied by**   **the available carbohydrate**
(divided by 100)   (in grams)

So – the GL of watermelon is 0.72 x 6 = 4.32, rounded to **4 GLs per 120g serving.**

So watermelon is high GI, but low GL – meaning it's good for you.

Here's another example showing why GL is a much more accurate way of gauging a food's effect on blood sugar than GI. Say you want to eat a carrot (up to 92 GI in some tables) and pumpkin soup (75 GI), followed by some salmon (neglible GI, as it's a protein), broad beans (79 GI) and sweet potato (44 GI in some books), followed by a slice of watermelon. You'd get a big tut-tut from the GI fanatics, who scorn any food above 70 GIs because it is fast-releasing, although you might get a mild brownie point for choosing sweet potato.

Now factor in the quantity of available carbs to get the (GL) for all these foods. Carrots (3.9 (GL)), pumpkin (4.3 (GL)), broad beans (4.1 (GL)) and watermelon (4.3 (GL) per 120g serving) all score low in the (GL) stakes because they don't contain a lot of carbohydrate. Conversely, the one apparently 'good' low-GI food – sweet potato – provides 17 (GL) per 150g.

So GI can be inaccurate. Put simply, GL is the best measure of whether a food, a meal, or a diet will help you achieve blood sugar control and lose weight.

Do you want to lose or maintain weight?

The Holford Diet is all about optimum health – energy and wellbeing – and weight loss is just one facet of this. This is why it's a diet for life.

When you follow the weight-loss diet, you will lose a steady 2lb (about 1kg) a week. The length of time you stay in this phase depends on how much you need to lose. It could be as little as four weeks, or up to three months. As this is eating for health rather than just shaving off the pounds, it's perfectly safe to stay in the weight-loss phase for longer if you need to.

You'll have a basic GL allowance of 40 during this weight-loss phase (plus an extra 5 (GL) for drinks or puddings). The GL of each recipe is clearly marked and we've provided sample menus to make getting used to this easy. Once you achieve your goal, you just keep eating the same foods, but increase your basic GL allowance to 55 (GL) (plus an extra 10 (GL) a day for drinks and puddings). So how might a typical day's menu for either plan look?

The weight-loss day

Breakfast, lunch and dinner each total 10 (GL), and you'll add in 5 (GL) per snack for two snacks to make the 40 (GL) total. (We've left out the 5 (GL) for drinks or puddings for the moment as they're dealt with on page 32.)

So you might start with Plum yoghurt crunch and a couple of slices of toasted rye bread with pumpkin seed butter for breakfast (10 (GL)); go on to elevenses – a punnet of strawberries (4 (GL)); have Greek salad with quinoa for lunch (10 (GL)); stop for a teatime snack of Thai mushroom broth (4 (GL)); and feast on Venison sausage and mixed pepper casserole with Sweet potato and carrot mash for dinner (12 (GL)). 'Free' drinks for the day include unlimited herbal teas, water, coffee substitutes and one diluted glass of juice.

If it looks painless – and downright delicious – that's no more than the truth, as you'll see when you get to the full menus and recipes in Part 2.

The maintenance day

Let's say you've reached your target weight. Your three main meals now clock in at 15 (GL) each, while snacks still total 10 (GL) for a total of 55 (GL). (Again, we've left out the 10 (GL) for drinks and puddings for the moment as they're dealt with on page 32.) Taking the same one-day menu as above, you'd be able to add in a dessert (say, Blueberry pancakes or a Baked apple with almond custard) and a glass of wine.

Carb mix and match

The menus on page 16 are just one idea. Given the number of recipes (and potential for improvisation and invention), the possibilities are endless. In the end, how you achieve the ⓖ in your day is up to you.

First, there's balancing the number of ⓖ. The main meal recipes are all in the 8 to 12 ⓖ range, for instance. So if you have an 8 ⓖ lunch, you can have a 12 ⓖ dinner, and vice versa. Then there are the types of low-GL carbohydrates you might want to eat. Depending on the meal you're having, you might want to split the 10 ⓖ quota per meal (using the weight-loss allowance as an example) across two different types of food. Here are three examples of how to do it.

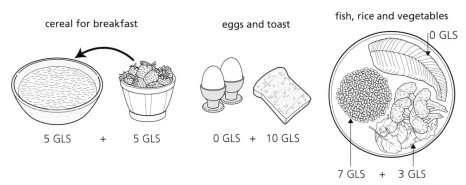

cereal for breakfast

5 GLS   +   5 GLS

eggs and toast

0 GLS + 10 GLS

fish, rice and vegetables

0 GLS

7 GLS   +   3 GLS

ⓖ, exercise and height

If you're keen on exercise, you might find that during the weight-loss phase, 45 ⓖ don't fill you up. The same also applies if you're very tall, while the reverse applies if you are very short. The chart below can help you adjust your ⓖ to fit your circumstances.

ⓖ PER DAY	Average exercise per day (mins)						
Height	0	15	30	45	60	90	120
5 ft (1.52m)	35	35	40	45	45	50	55
5 ft 3 (1.60m)	40	40	40	45	50	55	60
5 ft 6 (1.67m)	40	40	40	45	50	55	60
5 ft 9 (1.75m)	40	40	45	50	55	60	65
6 ft (1.83m)	45	45	50	55	60	65	70
6 ft 3 (1.91m)	50	50	55	60	65	70	75
6 ft 6 (1.98m)	55	55	60	65	70	75	80

Now let's sample the kind of carbohydrates you'll be eating the most of – low in ⓖ, but big on flavour, nutrition and versatility. In all the examples below, we use the weight-loss parameters of 10 ⓖ per meal and 40 ⓖ (excluding drinks and puddings) overall.

The best cereals, breads and pastas

In this section we'll look at the wonderful range of low-GL cereals and grain products you'll have to choose from.

The best cereals

If you're a devotee of cereal in the morning, your breakfast will look like this: a low-GL cereal, a low-GL fruit as a sweetener, and a source of protein and essential fats, such as yoghurt and seeds. The GL goal for weight loss, remember, is no more than 10.

In the chart below you'll see how much of the following common cereals you can have to total 5 GL. That leaves 5 GL for the fruit. As you can see, the best 'value' in terms of how much you can eat are oat flakes, either cooked as in porridge or eaten raw, just as you would cornflakes.

CEREAL	5 GL
Oat flakes	75g
Low-GL granola	125g/1½ servings (see page 68)
Cinnamon apple porridge	125g before adding milk/1 serving (see page 68)
Low-carb muesli	90g/1 serving (see page 67) ·
All-Bran	25g
Unsweetened muesli	15g
Alpen	15g
Weetabix	1 biscuit
Sweetened, refined cereals	10g

The best breads

If you have a protein-rich breakfast like poached or scrambled eggs, an omelette or kippers for breakfast, you can use up your entire 10GL quota on bread. Here's how much you'd get in a serving.

BREAD	10 GL
Nairn's rough oatcakes	5 to 6 oatcakes
Fine oatcakes (no sugar added)	3 to 4 oatcakes
Rye 'pumpernickel' style bread	2 thin slices (50g)
Sourdough rye bread	2 thin slices (50g)
Rye wholemeal bread (yeasted)	1 slice
Wheat wholemeal bread (yeasted)	1 slice
White, high-fibre bread (yeasted)	less than 1 slice

As you can see, your best 'value' breads are oat cakes. Rough oat cakes such as Nairn's, which are sugar-free, are best, followed by fine oatcakes, again provided they contain no sugar. Next best are Scandinavian-style or German-style breads such as pumpernickel, sonnenbrot or volkenbrot. These breads are genuinely 'wholegrain' – you can actually see the entire grain in them, which means they are less processed and slower releasing.

Next best is sourdough rye bread made without yeast. (Yeasted bread is problematic because its carbohydrate breaks down into high-GL simple sugars when cooked.) Unlike the light, white, fluffy 'fake' breads we've been conditioned to eat, which are full of air, over-refined and nutritionally inferior, sourdough and the like are real breads, substantial, fibre-rich and delicious.

Real breads are better for two reasons. One is the way they're processed. They have far fewer additives, use coarsely ground flours and, in the case of sourdough, have no added yeast. All this keeps the GL score lower.

Also, some grains are better than others because of the type of carbohydrate they contain. Wheat and corn are high in a fast-releasing sugar called amylopectin, while barley and rye are higher in one called amylose, which is slower releasing. As we've seen with cereals, oats are best of all the grains. While the GL of wheat varies depending on what's done to it, oats are relatively similar in any shape or form. Whole oat flakes, rolled oats or oatmeal, as used in oatcakes, all have a low-Glycemic effect.[1]

The best pastas
High-protein diets banish most pastas, but wholewheat pastas, especially those containing egg, have a reasonably low GL.

The chart below shows how much you can eat to equal a 7 Ⓖ serving.

PASTA (dry weight)	7 Ⓖ
White vermicelli	40g
Wholemeal wheat spaghetti	40g
Pasta, wholemeal	40g
Egg fettuccine	35g
White durum wheat spirali	35g
White spaghetti	35g
Instant noodles	35g
Durum wheat spaghetti	30g
Maize gluten-free pasta	25g
Macaroni	25g
Rice noodles	25g
Udon noodles	20g
Corn pasta	20g
Gnocchi	15g
Brown rice pasta	15g

Luckily, wholewheat pasta made with egg is now available from health food shops in many forms, from spaghetti and macaroni to penne and fettucini. There are also many non-wheat pastas, which are great if you're allergic to wheat, but they tend to be higher in Ⓖ. So, again, go easy on the quantity.

Combine your pasta with a source of protein, such as tuna (more on this on page 26), and plenty of vegetables. If you allow 3 Ⓖ for the vegetables, that'll give you 7 Ⓖ for the pasta. (Note that if you're eating starchy vegetables such as sweet potato at a meal, this will generally take the place of a serving of bread or pasta – see also page 22).

The best fruits

Everyone now agrees that a healthy diet is strong on fresh fruit, as they're so rich in vitamins, minerals and antioxidants. The only drawback is that some fruits are also very high in fast-releasing sugars and can send your blood sugar levels sky-high. Dates are one example. A single date has the same effect on your blood sugar as a whole large punnet of strawberries!

If you're eating fruit as a snack, remember that the goal in the Holford Diet is to eat no more than 5 Ⓖ of it, whether you're eating it on its own or with protein – say, a handful of almonds or some pumpkin seeds (see page 26). Similarly, if you are eating fruit with your breakfast cereal, your goal is to have a 5 Ⓖ serving of the fruit along with the 5 Ⓖ of the cereal. The chart below shows you the approximate amount of each fruit that equals 5 Ⓖ, with exact amounts in grams to the right.

As you can see, the Ⓖ of fruits differ vastly. The best fruits for balancing your blood sugar and your waistline are any kind of berries, cherries, plums, grapefruit, oranges, melons, pears and apples. The worst are dried fruits and bananas. This is partly because some fruits, especially dried ones, have less fibre in them (and as I noted earlier, fibre in a food will help to slow down the release of its sugars), but mainly because different fruits have different kinds of sugar in them.

This doesn't mean, however, that you have to bypass bananas and dried fruits forever. It just means you need to limit them, using the chart as a guide, and ensure you do eat seeds or nuts – a source of protein – with them. Remember that it's vital to feel satisfied when you eat, and a punnet of cherries is bound to fill you up more than 10 raisins.

FRUIT	5 Ⓖ	in grams
Blackberries	1 large punnet	600g
Blueberries	1 large punnet	600g
Raspberries	1 large punnet	600g
Strawberries	1 large punnet	600g
Cherries	1 punnet	200g
Grapefruit	1 small	200g
Pear	1 large pear	150g
Melon/cantaloupe	1/2 a small melon	150g
Watermelon	1 big slice	150g
Peach (fresh or canned in natural juice)	1 peach	120g
Apricot	4 apricots	120g
Orange	1 large	120g
Plum	4 plums	120g
Apple	1 small	100g
Kiwi fruit	1 kiwi	100g
Pineapple	1 thin slice	85g
Grapes	10 grapes	75g
Mango	1 slice	75g
Tinned fruit cocktail	1/2 a small can	65g
Papaya, raw	1 slice	60g

Banana	½ small	50g
Tinned apricots (in light syrup)	⅓ small tin	50g
Tinned lychees (in syrup and drained)	⅕ 200g can	35g
Prunes	3 prunes	30g
Dried apricot	3 apricots	30g
Dried apple	3 rings	30g
Dried figs	1 fig	20g
Sultana	10 sultanas	10g
Raisins	10 raisins	10g
Dates	1 date	5g

On the whole, though, you'll be concentrating on low-GL fruit – and you'll hardly struggle to eat plums, berries, pears and watermelon! You can have them as snacks or in our delicious low-GL puddings. In any case, aim for two to three servings of fruit every day, for example two as snacks and one with breakfast or in a dessert.

See the table on page 33 for details on how much fruit juice you can drink on the Holford Diet.

The best vegetables

Just like fruit, not all vegetables are created equal. Some, such as potatoes, are richer in carbohydrate – the so-called starchy vegetables. Others, such as most salad vegetables, are very low in starch.

We recommend a combination of both in most main meals, allocating 7 ⓖⓛ for the starchy vegetables, which fill you up more, and up to 3 ⓖⓛ for the non-starchy vegetables. (Remember that the protein in the meal doesn't add to the GL count.) Our recipes calculate this for you.

What does this look like?

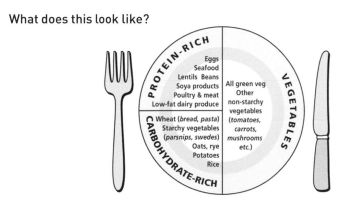

In sorting out how this will work, it can help to think of how much of what vegetable will cover your plate. Half the plate will hold non-starchy vegetables, and a quarter will be covered with carb-rich food, which might include starchy vegetables. The remaining quarter is for the protein-rich foods, such as chicken or fish.

Starchy vegetables

So your starchy veg and protein are around the same size – except where there's a big difference in how dense or weighty they are. So if you opt to eat chicken with squash, the serving size of squash is somewhat larger than the piece of chicken because chicken is dense and heavy, and squash is relatively light.

Let's take a look at the quantity of different starchy vegetables you can eat to keep within the 7 Ⓖ limit.

STARCHY VEGETABLES (uncooked weight)	7 Ⓖ
Pumpkin/squash	185g
Carrot	160g
Swede	150g
Beetroot	110g
Boiled potato	3 small potatoes (75g)
Sweet potato	1/2 sweet potato (60g)
Corn on the cob	1/2 a cob (60g)
Baked potato	1/2 baked potato (60g)
French fries	50g
Broad beans	30g

As you can see, there are some obvious winners. Swede, carrot and squash are much better GL value than potatoes. Boiled potatoes are better than baked, which are in turn better than French fries.

Some of these foods may be new to you – but all the more reason to give them a go! You'll be bowled over by the smooth, rich flavour of squashes, which are delicious mashed, baked or boiled.

Alternatively, instead of allocating 7 Ⓖ to a starchy vegetable, you might want to choose pasta or bread (see pages 18–19), or grains, beans or lentils (see pages 23–24).

Unlimited vegetables

Now it's time to move to the other half of your plate. This is made up of what we call 'unlimited' vegetables. Sounds fabulous, doesn't it? Of course, there are limits, but most of these vegetables are so low GL that a serving can be really satisfying. A 2GL serving of peas, for instance, is a cupful.

We've allocated 3 Ⓖ for these non-starchy vegetables, so eat as much of them as you like, or can. The more you fill yourself up with them, the better you'll feel – and look – thanks to the vitamins, minerals and other phytonutrients they're brimming with. We've used them copiously in our recipes to keep you superhealthy.

UNLIMITED VEGETABLES

Asparagus	Endive	Radish
Aubergine	Fennel	Rocket
Bean sprouts	Garlic	Runner beans
Broccoli	Kale	Spinach
Brussels sprouts	Lettuce	Spring onions
Cabbage	Mangetout	Tenderstem
Cauliflower	Mushrooms	Tomatoes
Celery	Onions	Watercress
Courgette	Peas	
Cucumber	Peppers	

The best grains, beans and lentils

When it comes to grains, beans and lentils, most people in the West concentrate on wheat (in cereals, breads and pastas). Yet there's a positive cornucopia of amazing grains and beans out there to give your daily meals an entirely different and delicious taste and texture.

One of the best low-GL grains – although strictly speaking it's a seed – is quinoa, which hails from the Andes. Quinoa is also one of the best sources of protein in the plant kingdom. It boils just like rice but takes only 15 minutes to cook, and has a wonderful nutty taste. Here are some other grains you might like to try.

GRAINS (Dry weight)	7 GLs
Quinoa	65g
Cornmeal	60g
Pearl barley	45g
Bulgur	45g
Brown basmati rice	45g
Brown rice	35g
Buckwheat	30g
Instant white rice	30g
White basmati rice	25g
White rice	25g
Couscous	25g
Millet	20g
Whole rye kernels	15g
Whole wheat kernels	15g

The reason why some grains are better than others is because of the type of carbohydrate, or sugar, they contain. As we saw on page 19, wheat is high in a fast-releasing sugar called amylopectin. Quinoa and barley, however, are higher in amylose, which is slower-releasing. Most rice, by the way, has a high GL score because it contains a large proportion of amylopectin. Basmati rice, however, has more amylose and is therefore slower-releasing. Brown basmati is best. This is why brown basmati rice appears so often in this book – you can eat more of it.

The best beans and lentils

Beans and lentils, collectively known as pulses, are a true superfood. They're
superb for boosting your energy while helping you keep your weight steady.
How do they manage it? Pulses are a mix of both carbohydrate and protein,
and many contain naturally slow-releasing sugars anyway, all of which makes
them low GL. They also contain special phytonutrients that help to keep your
hormones in balance.

Pulses are incredibly versatile in other ways. You can use them either
as a main ingredient in a meal, providing both protein and carbohydrate,
or together with another carbohydrate food and protein food.

The bottom line is that they're all good for you, except for beans tinned
with loads of sugar. When you buy beans in tins, for example baked, cannellini
or kidney beans, buy the ones without added sugar. Any meal containing beans
and lentils can be quite generous with the portion size – remember, you're
getting both protein and the carbohydrate from the same food here.

However, when you are eating these foods as your source of protein,
combine them with only half the serving size of a carbohydrate-rich food,
instead of an equal serving. In practice, that means that if you're making our
delectable Lentil stew (see page 137), you'd have two parts lentils to one part
rice. This is, of course, because you're already getting a significant amount
of carbohydrate in the lentils.

The table below shows you how much you can eat to achieve 5 Ⓖ (if
you're eating them with another source of carbohydrate – rice and beans
for example), or 7 Ⓖ if they are your sole source of starchy carbohydrate in
the meal. (Most regular cans of beans provide around 225 to 245g of beans.)

BEANS AND LENTILS	5 Ⓖ (cans)	5 Ⓖ (grams)	7 Ⓖ (cans)	7 Ⓖ (grams)
Soya beans	3 1/2	750	4 1/2	1050
Peas	1 3/4	375	2 1/2	525
Pinto beans	1	187	1	262
Borlotti beans	1	187	1	262
Lentils	3/4	150	1	210
Butter beans	1/2	125	3/4	175
Split peas	1/2	125	3/4	175
Baked beans	1/2	107	3/4	150
Kidney beans	1/2	107	3/4	150
Chickpeas	1/2	94	1/2	132
Chestnuts	1/2	94	1/2	132
Flageolet beans	1/2	83	1/2	116
Haricot/navy beans	1/3	62	1/3	87
Black-eyed beans	1/3	58	1/3	81
Baked beans (low sugar)	1/3	57	1/3	80

The best snacks

The Holford Diet is all about enjoying your food while losing weight and boosting health, and snacks give you even more scope for enjoyment. But what to eat?

If your blood sugar or hormones are out of balance, you might have built up a sugar habit – reaching for a chocolate bar, say, when 11am strikes. But eating between meals isn't a bad thing at all. Research shows clearly that 'grazing' (eating little and often) is healthier for you than 'gorging' (having one or two big meals in the day),[2] as we'll see in more detail on page 29. Grazing helps keep your blood sugar levels even, and makes overeating far less likely, as you'll never experience any between-meal hunger pangs.

So you'll find that I recommend a mid-morning and a mid-afternoon snack. Of course, the key thing here is what you eat. The ideal snack provides no more than 5 GL and also some protein, and the simplest is fruit. See pages 20–21 for the table which provides 5GL amounts of a wide variety of fruit.

As we've seen, berries (whatever's in season, or frozen mixed berries), plums and cherries are your best-'value' fruit snacks. You can further slow down the GL score of these fruits by eating them with five almonds or a dessertspoon of pumpkin seeds. Other than chestnuts, almonds are the best nut because they have the most protein for their caloric value. Pumpkin seeds are also high in protein, and in beneficial omega-3 fats. Flax seeds are the highest for omega-3s, but are too small and too hard to make good snacks, so you'll need to grind them up.

Another snack option is protein-based spreads. Cottage cheese, hummus and sugar-free peanut butter are all excellent. Hummus, the popular Middle Eastern chickpea dip, is deliciously rich-tasting as well as low GL. You could have it with bread or oat cakes (see below), or a raw carrot – a large carrot is still less than 5 GL.

The table below shows the GL for all these spreads and dips, as well as the easy, incredibly tasty ones we've devised for this cookbook. Note that for dips, the snack serving size is about 150g – half a small tub of cottage cheese or supermarket hummus – while for spreads it's about a tablespoon. Have these dips with an oat cake or crudités, such as slices of carrots, peppers

DIPS/SPREADS	GL per serving
Hummus	1
Cottage cheese	1
Guacamole	1 (see p. 81)
Satay dipping sauce	1 (see p. 82)
Yoghurt satay dip	1 (see p. 80)
Avocado and cream cheese dip	2 (see p. 79)
Peanut butter	2
Creamy tahini dip	2 (see p. 79)
Hummus and egg pâté	2 (see p. 82)
Goat's cheese and artichoke pâté	3 (see p. 82)
Spicy Mexican bean dip	4 (see p. 80)
Roasted red pepper hummus	5 (see p. 83)

or tomatoes. Oat cakes contain beta-glucans, a type of fibre that helps to slow down the release of glucose into the blood, lessen insulin response and also lower cholesterol and heart disease risk. Of all the grains, oats are the best for losing weight, and for controlling your blood sugar.[3]

Watch out when buying oat cakes, though. As we've seen, the best are Nairn's. Not only do they make a sugar-free, organic version, but they also use palm fruit oil, which contains unsaturated fat, as opposed to palm oil, which is higher in saturated fat.

Here are some 5GL snacks to choose from – bearing in mind that these are only a few out of a huge selection:

SNACKS FOR 5 GL

- 1 piece of fruit, plus 5 almonds or a dessertspoon of pumpkin seeds
- Berries and *either* 1 small plain yoghurt (150g) *or* $\frac{1}{2}$ a small tub of cottage cheese (150g)
- 1 thin slice of rye bread or 2 oat cakes and *either* $\frac{1}{2}$ a small tub of cottage cheese (150g), $\frac{1}{2}$ a small tub of hummus (150g) *or* peanut butter
- Crudités (a carrot, pepper, cucumber or celery) and *either* $\frac{1}{2}$ a small tub of hummus (150g) *or* $\frac{1}{2}$ a small tube of cottage cheese (150g)
- 1 boiled egg with 2 oat cakes
- Any of the dips on page 25 with *either* 1 small carrot and celery crudités *or* 1 oat cake
- Greek salad skewers (see page 78)
- Antipasti skewers (see page 78)
- Hummus soufflé (see page 83)
- Gravadlax with quail's eggs (see page 85) on 1 small slice of rye toast
- Feta and olive roast peppers (see page 85)
- Thai mushroom broth (see page 87)
- Tamari toasted nuts (see page 79) and St Clement's smoothie (see page 182)

As you can see, you won't be bored between meals because of the huge scope for mixing and matching. You'll find the full array in Part 2.

GO FOR PROTEIN/CARB COMBINATIONS

Protein plays a vital role in the Holford Diet. Eggs, meat, fish and cheese help us lose weight because they have virtually no effect on blood sugar, yet fill us up. High-protein diets have shown us this, but they're problematic. High-protein diets, particularly those based on a high dairy intake, are associated with increased risk of breast, prostate and colorectal cancers. We need the phytonutrients that good-quality carbohydrates offer, in short.

So the best way to go is to eat protein with the kind of low-GL carbohydrates we've been exploring. That way, you stabilize blood sugar, feel less hungry, lose more weight – and stay optimally healthy.

The perfect balance is 60g of protein and 120g of low-GL carbohydrate divided evenly among your meals – that is, 20g of protein and roughly 40g of carbohydrate three times a day. The recipes we've devised will do this for you, and provide a template for you to use when you launch your own creations.

So for lunch or dinner eat a protein-rich food with an equivalent-sized serving of any starchy carb-rich food, plus a large salad or two servings of 'unlimited' (see page 23) non-starchy vegetables.

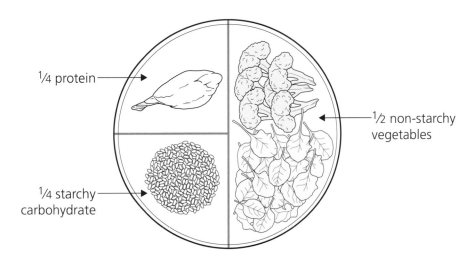

¼ protein

½ non-starchy vegetables

¼ starchy carbohydrate

How big is a protein serving?

PROTEIN	SERVING (in grams)	
Tofu and tempeh	160g	¾ packet
Soya mince	100g	3 tbsp
Chicken (no skin)	50g	1 very small breast
Turkey (no skin)	50g	½ small breast
Quorn	120g	⅓ pack
Salmon and trout	55g	1 very small fillet
Tuna (canned in brine)	50g	¼ tin
Sardines (canned in brine)	75g	⅔ tin
Cod	65g	1 very small fillet
Clams	60g	¼ can
Prawns	85g	6 large prawns
Mackerel	85g	1 medium fillet
Oysters	–	15
Yoghurt (natural, low fat)	285g	½ a large tub
Cottage cheese	120g	½ a medium tub
Hummus	200g	1 small tub
Skimmed milk	440ml	about ¾ pint
Soya milk	415ml	about ¾ pint
Eggs (boiled)	–	2
Quinoa	125g	1 large serving bowl
Baked beans	310g	¾ tin
Kidney beans	175g	⅓ tin
Black-eyed beans	175g	⅓ tin
Lentils	165g	⅓ tin

STARCHY CARB SERVINGS (dry weight)	7 GLs
Pumpkin/squash	185g
Carrot	160g
Swede	150g
Quinoa	65g
Beetroot	110g
Cornmeal	60g
Pearl barley	45g
Wholemeal pasta	40g
White pasta	35g
Brown rice	35g
Brown basmati rice	45g
White rice	25g
Couscous	25g
Broad beans	30g
Corn on the cob	½ a cob (60g)
Boiled potato	3 small potatoes (75g)
Baked potato	½ (60g)
French fries	50g
Sweet potato	½ sweet potato (60g)

What you'll probably find is that you'll be eating more protein in relation to your carbs, and more fruit and veg, than you're used to. (It makes a nice change to eat more, not less, and still lose or maintain weight!)

Winning combinations for main meals

PROTEIN	CARBOHYDRATES	VEGETABLES
Chilli con carne (see page 99)	on brown basmati rice	with a green salad
Marinated tofu	on wholewheat pasta	with steam-fried vegetables
Grilled chicken breast	and boiled new potatoes	with steamed runner beans
Cottage cheese	on oat cakes/rye bread	with broccoli and tomato salad
Venison sausages	and Sweet potato and carrot mash (see page 154)	with Roasted vegetables (see page 150)
Spiced turkey burgers	and Avocado potato salad (see page 151)	with Steamed Savoy cabbage with crème fraîche (see page 148)
Poached salmon	with Roast butternut squash with shallots (see page 153)	with Lemon and mint petits pois (see page 149)

As we've seen, protein/carb combinations are just as easy to put together for snacks and breakfasts. For instance, a few almonds or pumpkin seeds with a low-GL fruit slow the effect of fruit sugars on your blood sugar. And at breakfast, seeds, yoghurt or skimmed or soya milk with your cereal and fruit will achieve the crucial balance – whereas if you have egg on toast or kippers and oatcakes, you've done it already.

But remember – you don't have to take the DIY approach here. Our recipes do all this for you, and you will get a feel for this way of eating much sooner than you might think.

GRAZE, DON'T GORGE

Ever tried to eat just one or two meals a day? Hellish, isn't it? And, as we've now discovered, it's not good for you, either. Grazing – spreading your eating throughout the day – has proven to be a much more efficient and pleasurable way to get your daily (GL). This way you can stay satisfied and free of those 'I'd kill for a muffin' moments, keep your blood sugar levels even, avoid overeating and control your weight.

Remember that if you're aiming to lose weight, you'll consume 40 (GL) in all (excluding drinks and puddings), broken down into 10 (GL) each for breakfast, lunch and dinner, and 5 (GL) each for your mid-morning and mid-afternoon snacks.

Here's how that might look over three days of sample menus.

	EXAMPLE DAY 1	EXAMPLE DAY 2	EXAMPLE DAY 3
BREAKFAST	Low-carb muesli with berries and milk/yoghurt	Scrambled eggs and mushrooms with 1 thin slice pumpernickel style rye bread, toasted	Cinnamon apple porridge with Rhubarb compote
MID-MORNING	Apple with 5 almonds	Pear and 50g pumpkin seeds	Feta and olive roast peppers
LUNCH	Leek and potato soup	Salade niçoise and Hazelnut yoghurt	Roasted chickpea and lemon taboulleh with a tomato, basil and red onion salad
MID-AFTERNOON	Peanut butter and sunflower seed muffin	Carrot and walnut cake	Apricot crunch
DINNER	Pesto crusted salmon with boiled baby new potatoes	Chicken satay wrap	Chicken curry with brown basmati rice and vegetables
DRINKS	Unlimited water, herbal teas and coffee substitute, plus 1 glass of diluted juice	Unlimited water, herbal teas and coffee substitutes, plus St Clement's smoothie	Unlimited water, herbal teas and coffee substitutes, plus 1 glass of diluted juice

As you can see, this is a substantial amount of food, paced well. And you need to eat it to lose or maintain weight!

The single biggest mistake you can make is not to eat breakfast. This is when your blood sugar is lowest. Many people make the mistake of starting their day with a cup of strong tea or coffee. This does satisfy immediate hunger, but sets up a cycle of craving for the wrong foods. If you eat a low-GL breakfast, you will be less hungry, and eat less, during the day – and lose more weight.

Your golden rule must be to eat before you get to that 'starving-hungry' moment when you choose the wrong food and go into eating overdrive. And that's where your two low-GL snacks pick up the slack after breakfast. As well as the snack options listed on page 25, there are other possibilities as long as you stick with 5 Ⓖⓛ for each snack: soups, salads, and even muffins and cakes to solve any energy slumps morning or afternoon.

Having a decent lunch and dinner is as important as going for a good breakfast. You'll be preparing the ground for the next day, allowing yourself to wake up refreshed rather than tired, with rock-bottom blood sugar and a desperate need for a massive kickstart from espresso or slabs of white toast with jam. Ideally, leave two hours between dinner and bedtime so your food can digest.

CHOOSE GOOD FATS, AVOID BAD ONES

If you believed conventional calorie theory, you'd think low-fat diets were best. But we now know that what needs to stay low is GL – and that the GL of your diet predicts weight gain much more accurately than its fat content.[4] It may seem counterintuitive, but some kinds of fats boost the body's ability to burn fat. These are the essential fatty acids, or EFAs.

EFAs – otherwise known as the omega fats – are nutritional powerhouses, literally enhancing health thoughout the body. Omega-3 and omega-6 EFAs are the best, followed by the omega-9s. In the boxes below you'll see where they're found and what they do.

Foods rich in omega EFAs	
Omega-3 family	Salmon, mackerel, herring, tuna and sardines; flax seeds, pumpkin seeds and walnuts; and their oils
Omega-6 family	Sunflower, sesame and pumpkin seeds and their oils; also safflower oil, evening primrose oil, corn oil, soya oil
Omega-9 family	Olive oil, almonds, walnuts

Family values: omega EFAs in action

Omega-3s are amazingly versatile. First, they keep extra weight at bay by making hormone-like substances called prostaglandins, which help to control our metabolism and our body's ability to burn fat. They also help to limit potential damage to your arteries from bursts of high blood sugar (which can happen when you're eating refined carbs or drinking too much alcohol). They calm inflammation. They reduce the risk of heart disease and of dying from a sudden heart attack by 50 per cent,[5] and also halve your risk of ever suffering from Alzheimer's disease.[6] So it won't surprise you to learn that one of their key roles is to keep brain and nerves up and running smoothly (DHA, an omega-3, is one of the brain's building blocks).

Omega-6s, meanwhile, ensure your skin stays healthy and maintain hormone balance, which is why so many women take them for PMS.

Omega-3s and omega-6s are both polyunsaturated, which simply means that their molecules are structured in a certain way. Omega-9, or mono-unsaturated fat, is also good for you, with olive oil a particularly rich source. A number of studies have found that switching from saturated to mono-unsaturated fats helps to stabilise blood sugar levels, improve insulin resistance and control diabetes.[7,8]

Not surprisingly, given their star quality, EFAs are the fats we recommend in our recipes. As for the rest, there are saturated fats – but they simply don't come near EFAs in the health stakes, and our recipes go light on them. The real baddies, however, are polyunsaturated fats that have been processed (hydrogenated) or fried, known as trans-fats. Heating can also make them go rancid or oxidise them, which means they can damage body cells. So the word on trans-fats is: don't go there!

Trans-fat foods to avoid

French fries
Fried or barbecued hamburgers
Deep-fried fish burgers and fish in batter
Deep-fried chicken nuggets
Sweets and cheap chocolate bars (with a low cocoa content and vegetable fats instead of cocoa butter)
Potato crisps and corn chips
Biscuits
Doughnuts
Margarine
Mayonnaise
Most commercial salad dressings

Unfortunately, many processed vegetarian foods are also high in these hydrogenated fats. Check the label of vegeburger or vegetarian sausage packets. If the label mentions 'partially hydrogenated vegetable oils', don't buy it.

Going for the omegas
Most of us are deficient in omega-3s, making it even more vital to get the huge range of benefits these fabulous fats offer. The Holford Diet provides four easy ways to get them into your daily menus.

BREAKFAST – A dessertspoon of seeds (half pumpkin, half flax is excellent, or you can mix in some sesame and sunflower, too) with your breakfast cereal, yoghurt or Low-GL Get Up and Go (see page 66). We also use seeds a lot in our breakfast recipes.

SNACKS – A dessertspoon of pumpkin seeds with fruit.

MAIN MEALS – A small serving of oily fish or a dessertspoon of pumpkin seeds on salad.

SALAD DRESSINGS – A dessertspoon of seed oil.

To get enough essential fats, you need to pick two of any of these options each day. Limit oily fish to three times a week – except tuna, which owing to its contamination with mercury should be an occasional treat.

Although the Holford Diet provides less fat than what people consume on average, the biggest difference between the average diet and the Holford Diet lies not in the quantity but the quality of the fat. Following the Holford Diet means that less than a third of the fat you eat is saturated, compared with the usual two-thirds.

Our recipes will take care of all this for you. The way you cook foods is also important – see pages 43–5 for our recommended methods.

OPT FOR THE BEST DRINKS AND PUDDINGS

A convivial glass of wine and delectable 'afters' aren't off the Holford Diet menu. In fact, the choice of drinks (hot and cold), including our own mouthwatering low-GL inventions, is broad – and you have more than 20 puddings to choose from.

On the weight-loss plan, your allowance for drinks, puddings and sweets is 5 Ⓖ, on top of the 40 Ⓖ for everything else. (On the maintenance diet, it's 10 Ⓖ on top of your total of 55 Ⓖ.) Those 5 Ⓖ could be a glass of juice or wine, a pudding or even some chocolate – just not all four on the same day.

Drink up

Cold drinks

The best drink is water – 2 litres, or 8 glasses, a day. Any herbal teas, coffee substitutes and juices you drink count towards this. You'll find it becomes second nature – not least because you'll feel much better in every way, including less hungry.

Fruit juices, whether concentrated or fresh, have a relatively high GL because the fibre in the fruits has been removed. The best is grapefruit juice, followed by apple juice, although even this should be drunk diluted. Here's how much you can drink for 5 Ⓖ

DRINK	5 GL
Tomato juice	1 pint
Carrot juice	small glass
Grapefruit juice, unsweetened	small glass
Apple juice, unsweetened	small glass, diluted 50/50 with water
Orange juice, unsweetened	small glass, diluted 50/50 with water; or the juice of 1 orange
Pineapple juice	1/2 a small glass, diluted 50/50 with water
Cranberry juice drink	1/2 a small glass, diluted 50/50 with water

Alternatively, you could go for the range of delicious low-GL drinks we've concocted for this book. You'll find delicious fruit smoothies, refreshing Gingerade and Lemonade and cocktail classic the Virgin Mary (page 184).

A good rule of thumb is to have no more than one glass of juice a day totalling no more than 5 GL a day.

Alcohol

Technically, pure alcohol doesn't have a GL score, but its effect on the blood is similar to sugar's. So if you want to lose weight, avoid it during the first two weeks to a month of the Holford Diet. Aqua Libra, Amé and other soft drinks made of natural ingredients with no added sugar are good alternatives if you remember to keep within the 5 GL rule.

After that, you can drink in moderation – either a small glass of good-quality wine, half a pint of beer or lager or a small shot of spirits, three times a week. Of these, the best is neat spirits, then white wine, red wine and finally beer. Beer has the highest carbohydrate content, double that of red wine and eight times that of white wine.

Hot drinks

It's best to reduce or avoid caffeinated drinks: they play havoc with your blood sugar, weight and energy. Luckily, you can find excellent herbal teas and coffee substitutes now. In any case, when diet alone leaves you fizzing with energy, you won't need stimulants!

You can reintroduce weak tea if you like when the time comes, and drink it from time to time, but coffee has several addictive substances in it. Reserve it for an occasional treat.

TOP TIP
If you're addicted to coffee, try Teeccino with some frothed milk and a touch of cinnamon. If you're addicted to tea, try Rooibosch (red bush) tea with milk.

Sugar and sweets

For a lot of people, kicking the sugar habit could prove a little tough, but your tastebuds will become acclimatised. Fruit will help when you crave something sweet. Once you're sugar-free, the odd sweet food is no big deal.

The best sugar-free alternative is xylitol (see page 187 in Resources), and that's what we use in our recipes. A natural sweetener found in many fruits and vegetables, such as plums, its GL score is a seventh that of sugar and half that of fructose.

SUGAR	5 GL
Xylitol	10 tsps (50g)
Blue agave cactus nectar	10 tsps (50g)
Fructose	5 tsps (25g)
Lactose	2 tsps (10g)
Sucrose	1 heaped tsp (7g)
Honey	1 tsp (6g)
Glucose	1 tsp (5g)
Malt	1 tsp (5g)

Puddings

If you can't finish a meal without craving something sweet, you'll need to break the habit or your blood sugar – and weight – will continue to seesaw. It takes only three days in most cases. After your initial stimulant- and sugar-free period, limit desserts to one a week (you can have more in the maintenance phase).

You'll find wonderful recipes in Part 2 that don't exceed 5 GL, yet still taste rich and delicious. A few have higher GL for those special treats and occasions, in which case you may have to sacrifice a snack, or have a light, low-GL lunch. So enjoy!

AVOID YOUR ALLERGY FOODS

Astonishing as it seems, one in three people now have hidden food allergies. These can cause weight to pile on, mainly by promoting water retention and bloating, and leave you feeling completely exhausted, too. Testing for allergy, once such a chore, is now dead easy and can be done using home-test kits (see page 187 in Resources).

If you are allergic to the usual suspects, you'll find that our recipes can be easily adapted to suit your particular needs. The Cook's Notes for each recipe show which allergies they take into account.

Note, too, that when you have an allergy test, the lab will give you clear instructions on what to eat or avoid. After three months of abstaining from the allergen, you may find you can tolerate it in small doses, or even that the allergy disappears completely. Other people may need to be careful about those foods all their lives. If you'd like to read up on allergies in more depth, see *The Low-GL Diet Bible* or *Hidden Food Allergies* (co-author Dr James Braly).

The usual suspects

The ten most common foods or food groups that people are allergic to are listed below, in descending order. Be aware that you only need to avoid these foods if you've actually been shown to be allergic to them.

1 Cow's milk
2 Yeast
3 Wheat
4 Gliadin grains
5 Eggs
6 Oats
7 Nuts
8 Beans
9 White fish
10 Shellfish

Let's look at the three most common allergy-provoking foods in detail.

Cow's milk

This is the most common food allergen, so you won't find it in many of our recipes. It's present in most cheeses, cream, yoghurt and butter and is hidden in all sorts of food, sometimes as 'casein', or milk protein. Its status as the number one allergen isn't surprising. Cow's milk contains hormones specifically geared to the needs of a young calf, not human beings. It's also a relatively recent addition to the human diet. It's doubtful that our ancestors were milking buffaloes! And approximately 50 per cent of people stop producing lactase, the enzyme that's needed to digest milk sugar, once they've been weaned. Is nature trying to tell us something? (However, it's not the milk sugar that causes the allergic reaction. It's the casein, the milk protein.)

Yeast

Yeast is the second most common allergen, and if you're sensitive to it you need to scout it out in stock cubes and processed food. As our recipes feature wholefoods and fresh ingredients, and avoid yeasted breads, this should be far less of a problem for you. I also recommend using Marigold's yeast-free vegetable stock cubes and bouillon powders.

If you've noticed you feel bad – sluggish, tired or blocked up – after eating bread, but fine after eating pasta, you may be allergic to the yeast, not the wheat, in bread.

Beer and, to a lesser extent, wine also contain yeast. If beer or wine leave you feeling worse than spirits, you may be yeast-sensitive. Does this mean you can't drink? Not at all. Just stick to spirits and champagne. The only guaranteed yeast-free alcoholic drinks are pure spirits such as vodka, while champagne is made by a double-fermentation process that means there's virtually no yeast in it. Since you won't be drinking much alcohol anyway, stick to spirits for the three months after your initial abstinence period (see page 33), so your body has a chance to 'unlearn' your allergy.

Sensible, moderate alcohol consumption is important for another reason. Alcohol irritates the digestive tract, making it more permeable to undigested food proteins. This increases your chances of developing an allergic reaction to anything, and it's why some people feel worst when they both eat foods they are allergic to and drink alcohol.

Wheat

As far as grain allergies go, wheat is the big culprit. It contains gluten, a sticky protein also found in rye, barley and oats. Gluten sensitivity occurs in about one in a hundred people, but is medically diagnosed in fewer than 1 in 1,000. However, there is something in gluten, called gliadin, which some people react to specifically. If you have had an allergy test, you'll know whether you are gluten-, gliadin- or wheat-sensitive.

If you are completely gluten-sensitive, you'll have to cut out wheat, rye, barley or oats. Excellent alternatives are rice, quinoa, buckwheat, millet and maize or corn (although some gluten-sensitive people do react to corn). From the GL point of view, quinoa is the best as it's very protein-rich. These days, you can find rice, corn and buckwheat breads and pastas in bigger supermarkets and good health food stores.

There is no gliadin in oats. If you are gliadin-sensitive, then you can eat oats, but not wheat, rye or barley.

If you are only wheat-sensitive, it's relatively easy. Just eat rye, barley or oats. In our recipes simply substitute the grains you can eat, if you know you're allergic.

In conclusion . . .

The Holford Diet is the easiest, most effective and safest way to lose and maintain weight because it works with your body's design, not against it. Once you've embarked on the diet, you'll quickly find that your energy goes up, the pounds fall off, and you start – and end – the day glowing. Now you know the rules for low-GL eating, the next step is to learn how to prepare delicious meals that satisfy your tastebuds as well as your body's needs.

These recipes are all tried, tested and easy. They'll introduce you to new low-GL foods and you'll learn a range of simple tricks for making fast meals that are good for your waist and your health. They're versatile enough to work as a diet for life – and for everyone in your life.

Bon appétit!

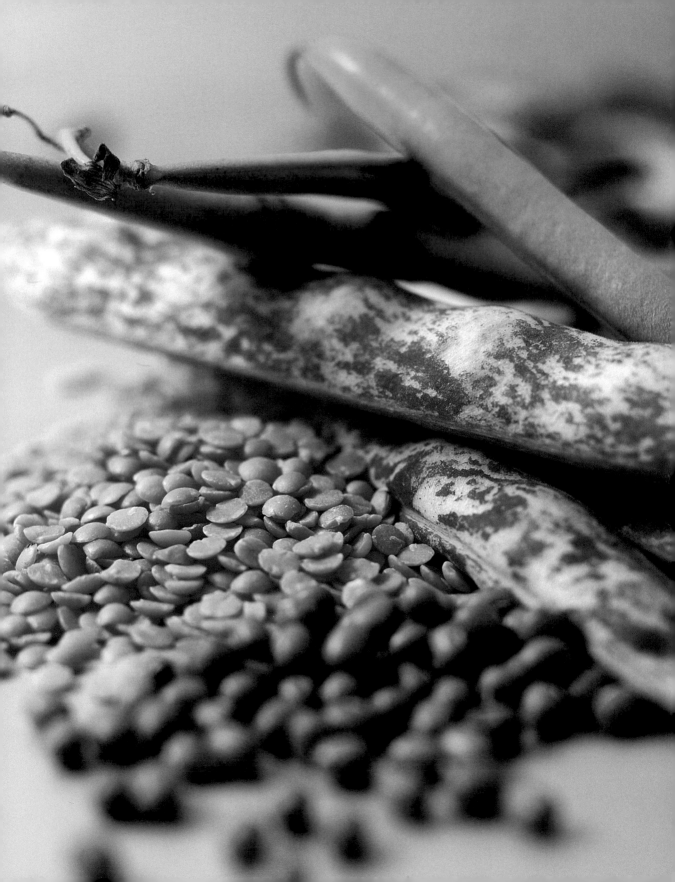

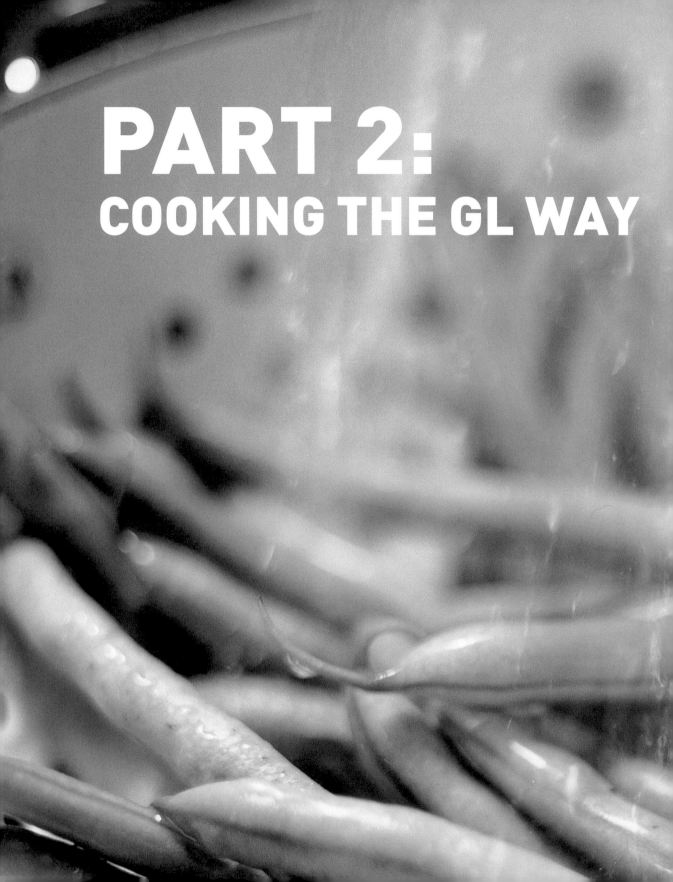

PART 2:
COOKING THE GL WAY

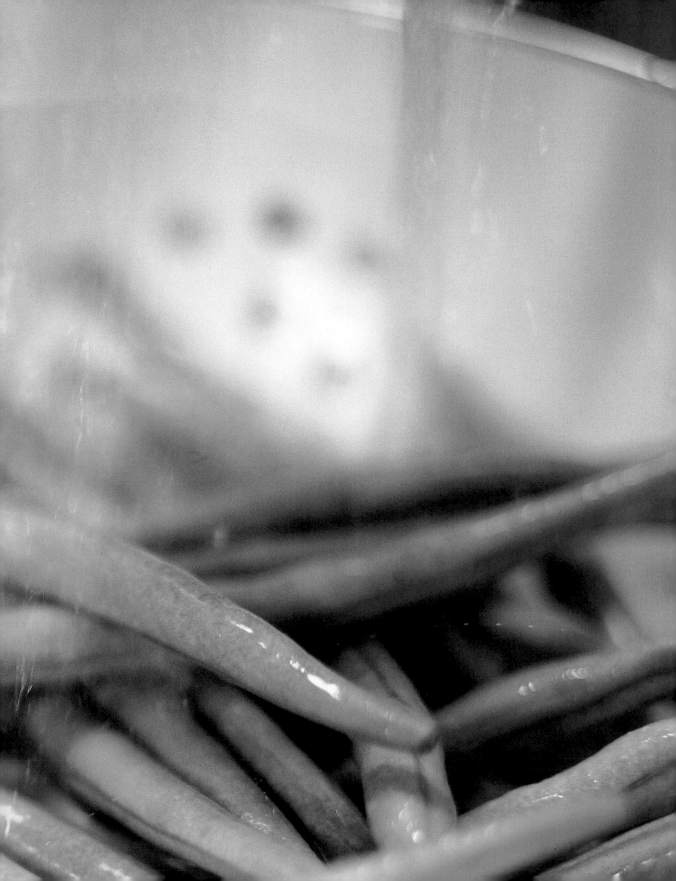

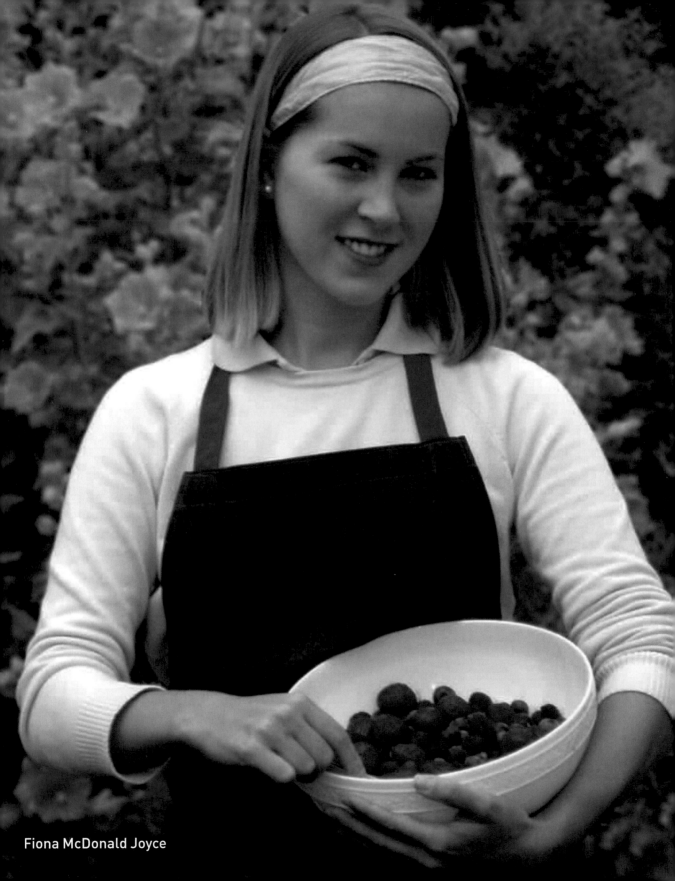

Fiona McDonald Joyce

GETTING STARTED

The recipes that follow are born of a love of good food coupled with a desire to eat healthily. Unlike the meals found in most diet books, these are to be enjoyed, not just endured. They'll appeal to everyone, and thanks to this, you won't have to make separate diet-friendly dishes for yourself if you are feeding friends or family as well.

Not only will these recipes make your day, tastewise, while helping you glow with wellbeing and lose weight into the bargain. They're also a doddle to cook. Like everyone else, we want meals that can be thrown together in minutes to fit in with our busy lifestyles. Even if you think you're not the world's greatest cook, you'll find them extremely easy.

In this part we'll go over everything you need to follow the diet. First, a word on how the recipes work; then, equipping your kitchen and buying your raw materials (neither of which will break the bank, or try your patience); then menu plans for both weight loss and maintaining your weight; and finally, the recipes themselves.

How it works

For weight loss

If you're wondering how to apply the GL principles I laid out in Part 1, just look at the Cook's Notes in the margin next to each recipe.

These show the ⓖⓛ for each serving, and the total ⓖⓛ per serving when accompaniments such as brown rice are added. You'll find suggestions for serving the dish, variations and allergy advice – although bear in mind that the allergy status of each recipe is based on the ingredients in it, not on the serving suggestions. Where appropriate, we have given alternatives to common allergens like wheat and dairy in the recipes (such as soya or nut milk), and as a result have rated the dish as dairy free, for example.

Remember, a day's worth of ⓖⓛ (including drinks or puddings) is 45 if you want to lose weight, so it's a simple matter of totting up the ⓖⓛ per dish to make your daily quota. To get you started, we have worked out a four-week menu plan for weight loss (pages 52–9).

Keeping track yourself

Once you get going, you can keep track of your ⓖⓛ by simply using the recipe margin notes and, if you need to, the GL tables for snacks – whether savoury (page 77), sweet (page 161), or simply fruit (pages 20–1) with nuts or seeds – as these will take up 10 ⓖⓛ in total each day. (Note that I've periodically included smoothies as snacks in the menu plans, although they appear in the Drinks section in this book.)

And, although the recipes tell you this, if you want guidance on serving sizes of carbohydrate foods for either weight loss or maintenance, you'll find handy tables for that on pages 19 and 23.

On to the maintenance phase

What about the transition from the weight-loss phase to maintenance? Remember, you'll be switching from a total of 45 to 65 ⓖⓛ a day. I'll be discussing what that means in real terms later on, but we've made it very easy to put into practice: just check out the tips on tailoring each dish to your maintenance needs in the margin next to each recipe, and have a look at the two-week maintenance menu plan on pages 62–3.

I promise that it will all start becoming second nature to you within a week. We've had great fun eating our way through all of the dishes here in the name of research. We think they're delicious and we really hope you enjoy them too, as they help you to lose weight and feel fantastic.

Equipping your kitchen

These recipes are designed to be as simple as possible. In fact, most of them were created and tested on Fiona's 28-foot boat, which has a microscopic galley and no fridge. So there is no excuse for crying off the cooking because of a lack of copper pans or other fancy kitchen paraphernalia – you won't need them!

Having said that, we would recommend that you have a saucepan with a steamer insert and lid, or an electric food steamer, as well as a wok with a lid for steam-frying (see below). Stainless steel pans are preferable to non-stick ones, as the non-stick coating can leach off and contaminate your food.

A handheld blender is a good idea for blending soups and making smoothies – or invest in the countertop kind, or a food processor, and you'll also be able to make delicious sauces like Pumpkin seed pesto (see page 143).

And finally, what about investing in a flask and some sealable plastic containers? That way, you can bring low-GL soups, salads and snacks to work during the week. Think Greek, niçoise or smoked fish salads, chicken wraps, gazpacho for the summer, hot bean soups for the winter, scrummy cakes and muffins – there's enough choice to help you stick to your diet and enjoy every meal.

Cookery techniques

Now that you've got your kitchen in order, a word on cookery techniques.

Keeping the GL load of your diet down, and your blood sugar even, isn't just about what you eat, but also how you cook what you eat.

All carbohydrate foods release their carbohydrate somewhat faster once cooked. The longer you cook something and the higher the temperature, the faster-releasing the food becomes. It's therefore best to eat food as close to raw as possible.

This doesn't mean endless salads. You can steam, steam-fry, boil and poach food without cooking it to death. Next best is baking, grilling, sautéing and stir-frying. Worst is frying and deep-frying.

Steaming is the best way of cooking green, leafy, less starchy vegetables, since it preserves a lot of their vitamins and minimises any raising of GL. The method can be used with any food and is very successful with fish – but perhaps not ideal with starchy vegetables, which require longer cooking, or with red meat. Many different kinds of steamers are available, or you can improvise with a colander, pot and lid.

Boiling raises the GL of foods more than steaming, but less than baking. Changes can be kept to a minimum by using as little water as possible, keeping the lid on, and cooking the food as whole as possible. Also, eat all vegetables al dente – a little crisp, not soft.

Steam-frying figures large in *The Low-GL Diet Cookbook* because it adds loads of taste without compromising on health.

The great advantage of this style of cooking is that the lower temperature of steaming doesn't destroy nutrients to anything like the extent that frying does, and you use only a small amount of oil, if that. As with boiling and ordinary steaming, aim to keep veg al dente.

To steam-fry, use a shallow pan or a deep frying pan with a thick base and lid that seals well. You can steam-fry without oil by first adding two tablespoons of liquid to the pan – water, vegetable stock, soya sauce or a watered-down amount of the sauce you'll use for the dish. Once it boils, immediately add some vegetables, 'sauté' rapidly for a minute or two, turn the heat up, add a tablespoon or two more of the liquid and clamp the lid on tightly. After a minute, add the rest of the ingredients. Turn the heat down after a couple of minutes and steam in this way until cooked.

Or you can add a teaspoon to a tablespoon of olive oil, butter or coconut oil to the pan, warm it, add the ingredients and sauté. After a couple of minutes, add two tablespoons of liquid as above and clamp the lid on. Steam ingredients till done.

Poaching is covering the food in liquid, like water, milk or a flavoured broth, and simmering to gently cook it in the liquid. You can make delicious water-based sauces. For example, you could cook fish in vegetable broth flavoured with ginger, garlic, lemongrass, spices and wine (the alcohol boils off).

Waterless cooking requires specially designed pans in which you can 'boil' foods by steaming them in their own juice and 'fry' foods with no oil. Both methods are excellent for preserving both nutrients and flavour.

Baking is useful, especially if the food is large and has a thick skin (such as a whole or half pumpkin). Avoid coating food with oil, because the oil will oxidise with cooking, which creates free radicals (highly reactive, harmful molecules). You can roast a potato without adding oil. The higher the temperature and the longer you cook something, the higher the GL becomes.

Frying should be kept to a minimum, and deep-frying avoided altogether. When you do fry, use coconut oil (saturated fats) or olive oil (monounsaturated) rather than other vegetable oils (poly-unsaturated oils), since they are much less prone to oxidation.

Grilling foods that contain fat is less damaging than frying, but browning or burning a food does create free radicals. Try to avoid barbecued food, or at least ensure that what you eat is not charred.

Microwaving is a problematic cooking method, although admittedly fast. As food cooks in its own water, it seems better than most cooking methods for preserving the water-soluble vitamins B and C. A Spanish study, however, found that microwaved broccoli lost vast amounts of major antioxidants (nutrients working to rid the body of free radicals) compared with steaming. Moreover, the temperatures reached in fat particles are very high, so avoid microwaving oily fish: it will destroy the essential fats it contains. And remember that microwave ovens do give off electromagnetic radiation, even six feet away.

If you must microwave, it is better to use lower-voltage/heat settings for longer. Cover dishes to encourage steaming, although you do need to leave some room for steam to escape.

TOP TIPS
Buy foods as fresh and unprocessed as possible and eat them soon afterwards.
Eat more raw food. Be adventurous. Try raw courgette or beansprouts in salad.
Cook foods as whole as possible, slicing or blending before serving.
Use as little water as possible, preferably steaming, poaching or steam-frying.
Fry foods as infrequently as possible.
Favour slow-cook methods that introduce less heat.
Don't overcook, burn or brown food.

How to roast peppers

A number of snack and main-meal recipes in this book call for roasted red peppers. If you want to do your own rather than buy them from the deli or in jars, here's how you do it.

You can either spear each pepper whole on a long fork and hold it over a gas hob until the skin blackens, or, if you need to do several peppers, put them whole into a baking tin and bake for 20 minutes at 200C/400F/Gas mark 6. Cool the peppers in a bowl covered with clingfilm and peel off the skin, then remove the stem, seeds and bits of pith from inside.

What's in your basket?

Fresh fruits and vegetables

On average, about a gallon of herbicides and pesticides are sprayed on the fruit and veg that one person eats in a year. Shocking? Yes – and it's also a good reason to choose organic. Not only is organic produce relatively free of contaminants, it's also good value. Organic food has 26 per cent more 'dry' matter, and less water in it, than non-organic food grown with fertilizer. As a result, there's more to organic fruit and veg, and even though they may be more expensive you're actually paying for a more substantial product. And their mineral levels can be 100 per cent higher than those of non-organic produce.

Here are the kinds of fruit and veg you'll be putting in your basket:

- Fresh, low-GL fruits such as apples, pears, plums, apricots, berries
- Frozen mixed berries in bags. Berries have a very low GL and are full of bioflavonoids, and freezing them means you can eat them all year round
- Lemons, unwaxed if possible
- Fresh vegetables such as lettuce, rocket, watercress, spinach, cherry tomatoes, cucumber, spring onions, alfalfa sprouts, cress, courgettes, red and yellow onions, shallots, mushrooms, tenderstem broccoli (or the purple sprouting or normal varieties), cabbage, aubergine and peppers
- Baby new potatoes. These have the lowest GL of all potatoes, as they are younger and smaller and so have not developed such high carbohydrate levels
- Sweet potatoes. These are very rich in the antioxidant vitamin betacarotene, which is vital for protecting your immune system
- Fresh herbs such as basil, flat leaf parsley, coriander and chives
- Garlic
- Fresh root ginger.

Foods for your fridge

You don't have to wave goodbye to cheese or butter on the Holford Diet. You just need to pick the right kind and use them to best effect. Fresh fish, tofu and chicken, as well as omega-rich seeds, nuts and seed butters, can also find a good home in your fridge. Once again, go for organic wherever possible. This is particularly important with milk products, chicken and other meat, and soya products (soya is often genetically modified).

Here are the types of goodies you'll be stocking your fridge with:

- Skimmed milk or a dairy-free alternative such as soya, almond or hazelnut, or quinoa 'milk'. (Note that all these contain protein, lowering the GL; rice milk, however, is very high in carbohydrates and has a high GL, so avoid it)
- Low-fat cottage cheese and cream cheese, as well as feta, halloumi and soft mild goat's cheeses. Butter is useful occasionally, and keeps for a while
- Live natural yoghurt. Live sheep's or goat's yoghurt is more easily digested than cow's, and some people allergic to cow's can happily eat them
- Tofu (soya bean curd, which comes smoked, plain or marinated and ranges from very soft or 'silken' to very firm) or tempeh (fermented soya bean curd)
- Anchovies in olive oil fresh from the deli. Small oily fish like anchovies accumulate less pollution and fewer heavy metals than big carnivorous fish like tuna and swordfish, making them a safer source of omega-3 fish oils
- Fresh sardines – another small fish rich in omega-3s and low in contaminants
- Fresh free range (and organic) chicken
- Unsalted, unroasted nuts and seeds for snacking and cooking. These aren't from the chill cabinet but should be stored in your fridge. Go for sunflower, pumpkin, sesame and flaxseeds or linseeds, and any kind of nuts – Brazils are full of selenium, and they're all delicious
- Pumpkin seed butter. This needs to be refrigerated after opening to protect the delicate omega-3 and omega-6 fats it contains. It tastes very similar to peanut

butter but is richer in essential fats and zinc, and is a good alternative for most people with nut allergies.

Store-cupboard staples

Some of the foods that will find a home in your kitchen cupboards may be unfamiliar to you at this point – quinoa, mirin or soba noodles, for instance. Think of this as adventures in good eating: part of the fun of the Holford Diet is exploring parts of the supermarket you may have sailed past until now.

A good supermarket will stock almost all of these items. You may find that a few are kept in the speciality section; if you can't find them there, try your local health food store. Rest assured, however, that nothing here is difficult to source or particularly pricey.

As always, go for organic wherever possible.

- Organic or free range eggs. These are preferable from the point of view of taste, the welfare of the chickens and your own health. Eggs can be an excellent source of B vitamins, zinc, iron and phospholipids – fats required for cell membranes and a healthy brain – but they are only as good as the food the chicken was fed on. Look out for eggs from chickens fed on flaxseeds, a good source of omega-3 oils
- Dried or canned legumes and pulses. Lentils, chickpeas, beans such as borlotti, kidney and flageolet, and canned mixed pulses are all good. If you go for tinned, choose the ones canned in water, or rinse thoroughly before use to remove as much salt and sugar as possible
- Rye bread – pumpernickel style or sourdough. Anyone avoiding wheat should check labels carefully as some brands add wheat
- Rough oat cakes. These have a satisfyingly coarse and chewy texture and a lower GL than finely milled varieties
- Wholemeal pasta. Choose a gluten-free variety such as brown rice or buckwheat pasta if necessary – buckwheat has a lower GL than rice or corn pasta
- Brown basmati rice – this has the lowest GL of all rices so is the only one we recommend on the Holford Diet. It has a nutty flavour and chewy texture and is far more interesting than plain white rice
- Soba noodles, made from gluten-free buckwheat. These noodles cook very quickly and can be used hot or cold in salads and steam-fries or stir-fries. Look out for the 100 per cent buckwheat ones in supermarkets, as some brands also contain wheat
- Quinoa. This South American fruit, pronounced 'keen-waa', looks and cooks like a grain and is very similar to couscous. It contains all the essential amino acids, making it a perfect protein food, and it's also low in fat and rich in minerals
- Whole organic oats
- Whole barley and rye flakes. These can be used in place of oats, although they need slightly more cooking time
- Low-GL Get Up and Go. A delicious superfood smoothie mix, that you blend with fruit. See Resources page 187
- Cornflour for thickening sauces and puddings
- Coconut oil, a very stable oil for cooking. It's virtually flavourless and can be used for spreading, frying and baking – it is solid at room temperature and melts when heated to form an oil. It will not raise cholesterol or produce harmful trans-fats

when cooked. If you have difficulty obtaining it you can buy it from Totally Nourish – see Resources page 187

- **Extra virgin olive oil for salad dressings**
- Sesame oil for Oriental dressings and dishes and to enliven couscous, quinoa or rice salads
- **Mirin, or Japanese rice cooking wine**
- **Tamari, a wheat-free soy sauce**
- **Tahini, or ground sesame seed paste**
- Canned chopped tomatoes, tomato purée and sun-dried tomato paste. Cooked tomatoes contain more of the antioxidant lycopene than raw ones, making these a really healthy addition to meals
- **Mixed antipasti, preferably in olive oil. Try roasted peppers and sun-blush tomatoes**
- Marinated artichoke hearts in oil and canned artichoke hearts. Artichokes are good for the liver, aiding detoxification
- **Olives. Avoid any that list colourings and additives on the label. Greek Kalamata olives are wonderfully moist and full of flavour**
- Crunchy peanut butter (choose a sugar-free brand). Peanuts are fairly high in saturated fat and low in healthier polyunsaturated fats, but peanut butter is a useful store-cupboard ingredient for a number of recipes like satay sauce
- **Xylitol, a naturally sweet, low-carb sugar alternative that doesn't disrupt blood sugar levels and has a third of the calories of sugar. This is available from Totally Nourish – see the Resources section on page 187**
- Vanilla and almond extracts. Be sure to get extracts rather than artificial flavourings – these are full of chemicals and not the same thing at all. You can find them in the home baking section of your supermarket
- **Good-quality dark chocolate (around 70 per cent cocoa solids), such as Green and Black's. This kind is low in sugar and contains iron and magnesium plus the antioxidant procyanidin, which helps maintain heart health**
- Black peppercorns. You'll notice that pepper appears in most savoury recipes here, as it contains a substance that actually helps you digest your food
- **Low-sodium salt, or sea salt, to be used in moderation**
- Marigold Reduced-salt Vegetable Bouillon powder. This delicious, full-flavoured alternative to stock cubes is suitable for vegans and is gluten, yeast and soya-free. It can also be added to dishes at any stage of cooking; there is no need to dissolve it in water like stock cubes. Many supermarkets now stock it
- **Dried herbs and spices, including herbes de Provence, mixed Italian herbs, oregano, chilli powder and chilli flakes, cayenne pepper, curry powder, and ground cumin, coriander, turmeric, paprika and nutmeg. Seek out organic herbs and spices that haven't been irradiated – check availability in your local health food store. Exposure to radiation, which ostensibly kills off harmful bacteria, can leave harmful free radicals in food**
- Good-quality anchovies and sardines tinned in olive oil.

Now that your kitchen is fully stocked, you're ready to do a little forward planning on the food front. In the next section you'll find useful menus for either weight loss or maintenance.

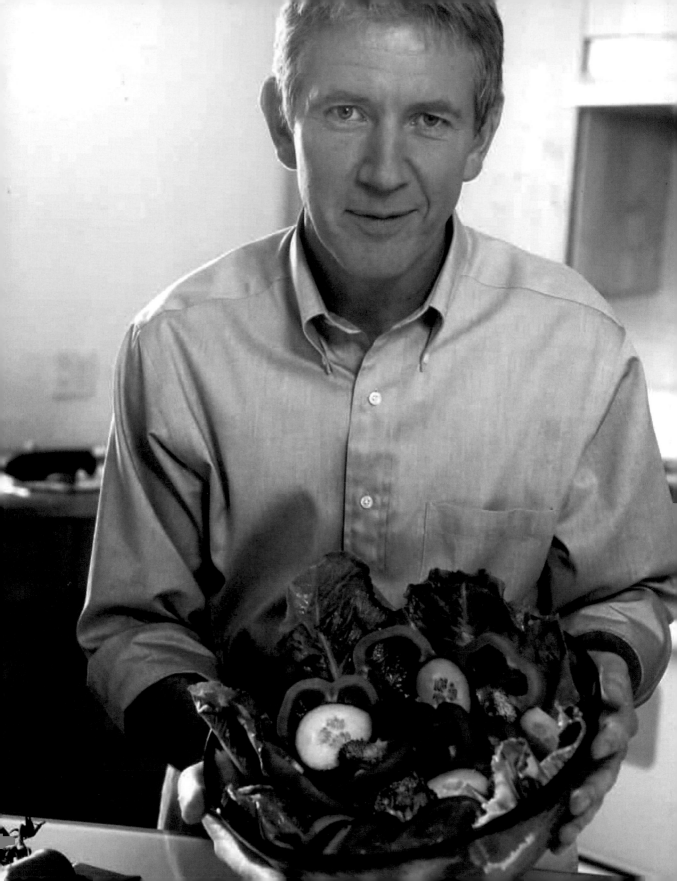

MENUS

Short of actually camping out in your kitchen to prepare your
meals, we have done all the hard work for you with this section.
The following menu plans – a four-week plan for weight loss, and
a two-week plan for maintenance – should get you off on the right
foot and help you get a real feel for the principles of low-GL eating.

But not just that: you'll begin to see how completely mouthwatering
these dishes are. Plum yoghurt crunch, Venison sausage and mixed
pepper casserole, Goat's cheese and artichoke pâté, Pear crumble
– with more than 150 recipes to try, there's enough variety to
thoroughly satisfy your tastebuds as you leave your old, sugar
-and-stimulant-fuelled life behind.

THE WEIGHT-LOSS PLAN

The following plan is designed to get you started on the Holford Diet weight-loss phase, giving you four weeks' worth of menus, and showing you how the GL points system works at each meal. However, these are simply our suggestions. You can adapt them accordingly, as long as you are having balanced meals that stick to your GL points allowance at the weight-loss stage. That's 45 Ⓖ, broken down as shown below.

Daily GL allowance for weight loss

Breakfast	10 Ⓖ
Mid-morning snack	5 Ⓖ
Lunch	10 Ⓖ
Mid-afternoon snack	5 Ⓖ
Dinner	10 Ⓖ
Additional points for drinks or puddings	5 Ⓖ
Total =	45 Ⓖ

If you are creating your own meal plans, you need to make sure that you are not getting too much or too little essential fat. This is about balance. So on the one hand don't shy away from them, and on the other don't have dishes full of nuts every day, avocado with every salad, or oily fish (such as salmon, trout, mackerel or fresh tuna) more than three times a week. In fact, it's now not advisable to eat the big carnivorous fish like tuna, swordfish or marlin more than once a month, owing to their contamination with high levels of mercury and other toxic metals.

WEIGHT-LOSS MENUS
WEEK ONE

Day 1
Breakfast Low-carb muesli with berries and milk/yoghurt
Lunch Leek and potato soup
Dinner Pesto crusted salmon with 3 boiled baby new potatoes, roasted cherry tomatoes on the vine and rocket
Snacks Apple with 5 almonds / Peanut butter and sunflower seed muffin
Drinks Unlimited water, herbal teas and coffee alternatives, plus 1 glass of diluted juice

Day 2
Breakfast Plum yoghurt crunch and 1 thin slice toasted rye bread or 1 medium slice wholemeal toast with peanut butter or pumpkin seed butter
Lunch Avocado gazpacho with sesame cornbread
Dinner Pork medallions with watercress salsa verde and 3 boiled baby new potatoes
Snacks Punnet of berries / Thai mushroom broth
Drinks Unlimited water, herbal teas and coffee alternatives, plus 1 glass of diluted juice

Day 3
Breakfast Scrambled eggs and mushrooms with 1½ thin slices toasted pumpernickel style rye bread or 1 medium slice wholemeal toast
Lunch Salade niçoise followed by Hazelnut yoghurt
Dinner Spiced turkey burgers with Sweet potato wedges and Red pepper and cucumber salsa
Snacks Pear and 1 dsp pumpkin seeds / Carrot and walnut cake
Drinks Unlimited water, herbal teas and coffee alternatives, plus St Clement's smoothie or 1 glass of diluted juice

Day 4

Breakfast Low-GL granola with Apple compote and milk/yoghurt
Lunch Chicken satay wrap
Dinner Roasted pepper and artichoke tortilla with rocket and watercress
Snacks 2 rough oat cakes with pumpkin seed butter or peanut butter / Pear and blueberry smoothie
Drinks Unlimited water, herbal teas and coffee alternatives, plus 1 glass of diluted juice

Day 5

Breakfast 2 boiled eggs and 1½ thin slices toasted pumpernickel style rye bread or 1 medium slice wholemeal toast
Lunch Stuffed pepper and green salad
Dinner Mediterranean tomato risotto with tuna and Baked fennel
Snacks Sesame and poppy seed muffin and Lemonade / Tahini yoghurt
Drinks Unlimited water, herbal teas and coffee alternatives, plus 1 glass of diluted juice

Day 6

Breakfast Cinnamon apple porridge
Lunch Roasted chickpea and lemon taboulleh with a tomato, basil and red onion salad
Dinner Chicken curry with brown basmati rice
Snacks Feta and olive roast peppers / Apricot crunch
Drinks Unlimited water, herbal teas and coffee alternatives, plus 1 glass of diluted juice

Day 7

Breakfast Smoked salmon and chive scrambled eggs on 1 medium slice wholemeal toast
Lunch Roast pepper and feta stuffed chicken with Sweet potato wedges and roasted courgettes
Dinner Smoked mackerel, leek and bean soup followed by Apricot amaretti biscuits
Snacks Antipasti skewers / Cheese platter
Drinks Unlimited water, herbal teas and coffee alternatives, plus a Virgin Mary or 1 glass of diluted juice

WEEK TWO

Day 1
Breakfast Low-GL Get Up and Go
Lunch Peter's Mediterranean bean feast with a large mixed salad
Dinner Feta and olive roast peppers followed by Moussaka with
a green leaf, tomato and basil salad
Snacks 2 apricots and 1 dsp sunflower seeds / Rhubarb fool
Drinks Unlimited water, herbal teas and coffee alternatives,
plus Pear and blueberry smoothie or 1 glass of diluted juice

Day 2
Breakfast 2 boiled eggs with 3 rough oat cakes
Lunch Hot smoked trout with pumpkin seed pesto and watercress open
sandwich followed by Tahini yoghurt
Dinner Chicken with cherry tomatoes and crème fraîche with half
a baked potato
Snacks Apple and 4 walnut halves / Peanut butter and sesame seed muffin
Drinks Unlimited water, herbal teas and coffee alternatives,
plus 1 glass of diluted juice

Day 3
Breakfast Low-GL granola with Rhubarb compote and yoghurt
Lunch Oriental chicken broth followed by Bresaola and artichoke
hearts on rye bread
Dinner Sun-dried tomato and black olive pesto with 55g wholemeal
pasta (dry weight) and a large rocket and red onion salad
Snacks Punnet of berries / Creamy tahini dip and crudités
Drinks Unlimited water, herbal teas and coffee alternatives,
plus St Clement's smoothie or 1 glass of diluted juice

Day 4

Breakfast Low-carb muesli with 2 chopped apricots and milk/yoghurt
Lunch Chestnut and butterbean soup
Dinner Chilli con carne with Sesame cornbread
Snacks Apple and 1 dsp pumpkin seeds / Hummus and egg pâté on 1 rough oat cake
Drinks Unlimited water, herbal teas and coffee alternatives, plus 1 glass of diluted juice

Day 5

Breakfast Scrambled eggs and mushrooms on 1½ thin slices toasted pumpernickel style rye bread or 1 medium slice wholemeal toast
Lunch Greek salad with quinoa
Dinner Thai mushroom broth followed by Red lentil and smoked mackerel kedgeree with steamed fine green beans
Snacks 1 small yoghurt with blueberries / Pear and 3 Brazil nuts
Drinks Unlimited water, herbal teas and coffee alternatives, plus 1 glass of diluted juice

Day 6

Breakfast 2 thin slices toasted pumpernickel style rye bread with pumpkin seed butter or peanut butter
Lunch Sun-blush tomato and black olive chickpea salad with Sesame cornbread and a green salad
Dinner Venison sausage and mixed pepper casserole with half a baked potato
Snacks Cottage cheese on 2 rough oat cakes / Apricot amaretti biscuits
Drinks Unlimited water, herbal teas and coffee alternatives, plus a Virgin Mary or 1 glass of diluted juice

Day 7

Breakfast Cinnamon apple porridge
Lunch Lemon and coriander chicken en papillote with brown basmati rice and steam-fried broccoli with garlic
Dinner Creamy salmon with leeks and steamed sugarsnap peas
Snacks Spicy Mexican bean dip with 1 rough oat cake / Thai mushroom broth
Drinks Unlimited water, herbal teas and coffee alternatives, plus 1 glass of diluted juice

WEEK THREE

Day 1

Breakfast Low-carb muesli with 1 small grated apple and milk/yoghurt
Lunch Cashew and sesame quinoa followed by Apricot amaretti biscuits
Dinner Halloumi and aubergine curry with brown basmati rice and a tomato and red onion salad
Snacks 2 plums and 5 almonds / 1 thin slice rye bread with pumpkin seed butter or peanut butter
Drinks Unlimited water, herbal teas and coffee alternatives, plus 1 glass of diluted juice

Day 2

Breakfast Cinnamon apple porridge
Lunch Aubergine pâté with 2 rough oat cakes and a rocket or watercress salad
Dinner Sesame chicken and soba noodle steam-fry
Snacks 2 apricots and 1 dsp sunflower seeds / Sesame and poppy seed muffin and Gingerade
Drinks Unlimited water, herbal teas and coffee alternatives, plus 1 glass of diluted juice

Day 3

Breakfast 2 poached eggs on 1½ thin slices of toasted pumpernickel style rye bread or 1 thick slice wholemeal toast
Lunch Chicken satay wrap
Dinner Tuna steak with sesame quinoa and a green salad
Snacks Apple and 4 walnut halves / Feta and olive roast peppers with 1 rough oat cake
Drinks Unlimited water, herbal teas and coffee alternatives, plus 1 glass of diluted juice

Day 4
Breakfast Low-GL Get Up and Go
Lunch Feta and flageolet bean salad with a Romaine lettuce salad,
followed by Almond custard
Dinner Spaghetti Bolognese
Snacks Apple and 5 hazelnuts / Peanut butter and sunflower seed muffin
Drinks Unlimited water, herbal teas and coffee alternatives,
plus 1 glass of diluted juice

Day 5
Breakfast Low-GL granola and strawberries with milk/yoghurt
Lunch Stuffed peppers with a green salad
Dinner Chilli con carne with Sesame cornbread
Snacks Tamari toasted nuts and St Clement's smoothie / Thai mushroom broth
Drinks Unlimited water, herbal teas and coffee alternatives,
plus 1 glass of diluted juice

Day 6
Breakfast Smoked salmon and chive scrambled eggs on 2 thin slices
toasted pumpernickel style rye bread or 1 thick slice wholemeal toast
Lunch Greek salad on a bed of cos lettuce with 2 rough oatcakes
Dinner Nick's beefburger in 1 wholemeal pitta bread with Spicy Mexican
bean dip and lettuce
Snacks Pear and 1 dsp pumpkin seeds / Baked chocolate orange pot
Drinks Unlimited water, herbal teas and coffee alternatives

Day 7
Breakfast Low-GL granola with Rhubarb compote and milk/yoghurt
Lunch Chicken with aubergine and peppers with brown basmati rice
or half a baked potato
Dinner 55g wholemeal pasta (dry weight) with Pumpkin seed pesto
and a green leaf, tomato and red onion salad
Snacks Greek salad skewers / Tamari toasted nuts, plus Strawberry smoothie
Drinks Unlimited water, herbal teas and coffee alternatives,
plus 1 glass of diluted juice

WEEK FOUR

Day 1

Breakfast Low-carb muesli with 1 small grated apple and milk/yoghurt
Lunch Roasted pepper and artichoke tortilla
Dinner 2 good-quality lean sausages with Giant baked beans
and a mixed salad
Snacks 2 apricots and 1 dsp sunflower seeds / Hummus and egg pâté
with 1 rough oat cake and cress, alfalfa sprouts or cucumber slices
Drinks Unlimited water, herbal teas and coffee alternatives,
plus 1 glass of diluted juice

Day 2

Breakfast 2 boiled eggs with 3 rough oat cakes
Lunch Leek and potato soup
Dinner Teriyaki salmon with steam-fried vegetables and brown basmati rice
Snacks Apple and 4 walnut halves / Oriental chicken broth and Lemonade
Drinks Unlimited water, herbal teas and coffee alternatives,
plus 1 glass of diluted juice

Day 3

Breakfast 2 thin slices toasted pumpernickel style rye bread with
Pumpkin seed butter or peanut butter
Lunch Chicken satay wrap
Dinner Borlotti Bolognese with quinoa and a green salad
Snacks Pear and blueberry smoothie / Avocado and cream cheese
dip with 1 small carrot and celery crudités
Drinks Unlimited water, herbal teas and coffee alternatives,
plus 1 glass of diluted juice

Day 4
Breakfast Low-GL granola with 2 chopped fresh apricots and milk/yoghurt
Lunch Smoked venison, Parmesan and mushroom salad with 3 boiled baby new potatoes
Dinner Cauliflower dahl with brown basmati rice or half a baked potato/sweet potato
Snacks Creamy tahini dip on 1 rough oat cake / Thai mushroom broth and Gingerade
Drinks Unlimited water, herbal teas and coffee alternatives, plus 1 glass of diluted juice

Day 5
Breakfast Cinnamon apple porridge
Lunch Sun-blush tomato and black olive chickpea salad with Sesame cornbread
Dinner Bangers and mash
Snacks Yoghurt and blueberries / Goat's cheese and artichoke pâté on 1 rough oat cake
Drinks Unlimited water, herbal teas and coffee alternatives, plus 1 glass of diluted juice

Day 6
Breakfast Low-carb muesli with Apple compote and milk/yoghurt
Lunch Spiced turkey burgers with Guacamole and lettuce in 1 wholemeal pitta bread
Dinner Salmon and cherry tomato bake with 3 boiled baby new potatoes and a rocket salad
Snacks Apple and 3 Brazil nuts / 2 rough oat cakes with cottage cheese and cucumber slices, alfalfa sprouts or cress
Drinks Unlimited water, herbal teas and coffee alternatives, plus 1 glass of diluted juice

Day 7
Breakfast 2 poached eggs on 2 thin slices toasted pumpernickel style rye bread or 1 thick slice wholemeal toast
Lunch Grilled chicken breast or pork chop (fat trimmed) with Sweet potato and carrot mash and Steamed Savoy cabbage with crème fraîche
Dinner Chestnut and butterbean soup
Snacks Greek salad skewers / Apple and almond cake
Drinks Unlimited water, herbal teas and coffee alternatives, plus 1 glass of diluted juice

THE MAINTENANCE PLAN

Once you've achieved your target weight, you have even more to look forward to. As you increase your overall food and drink intake from 45 to 65 GL a day, you'll be adding in more carbs, although meals will still be low-GL. We've provided a couple of weeks' worth of menus in this section to show you how to maintain your weight, and guarantee that you don't ruin all your hard work.

You'll see how wonderfully simple it is to make low-GL eating a habit for life. For instance, you can eat more low-GL desserts if you like, such as Fiona's fabulous Baked chocolate orange pots. These may taste decadent, but they are actually a low-GL pud packed with nutrients – so you can feel smug while you indulge!

So your points allowance will now look like this:

	Daily GL allowance for weight maintenance
Breakfast	15 GL
Mid-morning snack	5 GL
Lunch	15 GL
Mid-afternoon snack	5 GL
Dinner	15 GL
Additional points for drinks and/or puddings	10 GL
	Total= 65 GL

By now your blood sugar should be well balanced, leaving you buzzing with healthy energy and better able to resist the call of the biscuit tin or coffee bar. So the increased points allowance is not carte blanche to re-introduce that mid-morning cappuccino or custard cream; rather, it's a means to sustain your new weight and energy levels and add a delicious extra dimension to the healthy eating you're now familiar with.

In terms of protein and carbohydrates, what the maintenance phase means in practice is that you will reduce your protein intake from 25 per cent of your daily calories to between 15 and 20 per cent, and up your carb quota. So your main meals will amount to 15 GL each. This can come from a 10 GL main course plus a 5 GL starter, pudding or drink, or from more brown basmati rice, sweet potato or other carb serving with the meal – it's up to you. You'll still eat two 5 GL snacks a day but will have an additional 10 GL for drinks and/or puddings a day.

If this sounds like you need to take your calculator to each meal, trust us: it's very straightforward. We have included maintenance phase carbohydrate serving sizes and menu options with each recipe, where appropriate, to make this as simple as possible. We are all different, however, with different builds, metabolisms and lifestyles, so you may need to experiment and adjust the protein: carbohydrate ratio to suit you in order to look and feel your best.

MAINTENANCE MENUS

WEEK ONE

Day 1
Breakfast Cinnamon apple porridge with Fruit salad
Lunch Roasted chickpea and lemon taboulleh followed by Marzipan truffles
Dinner Chicken with cherry tomatoes and crème fraîche with 1 small baked potato and green salad
Snacks Apple with 1 dsp pumpkin seeds / Creamy tahini dip with half a small carrot and celery crudités
Drinks Unlimited water, herbal teas and coffee alternatives, plus 2 glasses of diluted juice

Day 2
Breakfast Low-carb muesli
Lunch Greek salad on a bed of Romaine lettuce with 1 wholemeal pitta bread
Dinner Vegetable chilli with brown basmati rice
Snacks Punnet of berries / Thai mushroom broth
Drinks Unlimited water, herbal teas and coffee alternatives, plus 1 glass of diluted juice

Day 3
Breakfast Fruit salad and yoghurt followed by 1 thin slice pumpernickel style rye bread with pumpkin seed butter or peanut butter
Lunch Avocado gazpacho followed by Salade niçoise
Dinner Chicken with aubergine and peppers with wholemeal pasta followed by Lemon cheesecake
Snacks Hummus and egg pâté with crudités / Apricot crunch
Drinks Unlimited water, herbal teas and coffee alternatives, plus 2 glasses of diluted juice

Day 4
Breakfast Low-GL granola with Apple compote and milk/yoghurt
Lunch Peter's Mediterranean bean feast with 1 wholemeal pitta bread and lettuce
Dinner Wholemeal pasta with Anchovy and tomato pasta sauce and a green salad
Snacks Apple and 3 Brazil nuts / 1 boiled egg with 2 rough oat cakes
Drinks Unlimited water, herbal teas and coffee alternatives, plus 2 glasses of diluted juice

Day 5
Breakfast Cinnamon apple porridge with 1 thin slice toasted pumpernickel style rye bread with pumpkin seed butter or peanut butter
Lunch Feta and flageolet bean salad with quinoa and watercress
Dinner Spaghetti Bolognese followed by Pear and baked custard pudding
Snacks 2 apricots and 1 dsp sunflower seeds / Thai mushroom broth
Drinks Unlimited water, herbal teas and coffee alternatives, plus Virgin Mary and 1 glass of diluted juice

Day 6
Breakfast 2 thin slices toasted pumpernickel style rye bread with 2 poached eggs
Lunch Thai mushroom broth followed by Chicken satay wrap
Dinner Nick's beefburger in wholemeal pitta bread with Spicy Mexican bean dip and lettuce
Snacks Pear and blueberry smoothie / Tamari toasted nuts and Sesame and poppy seed muffin
Drinks Unlimited water, herbal teas and coffee alternatives, plus 2 glasses of diluted juice

Day 7
Breakfast Scrambled eggs and mushrooms with 1 grilled tomato on 1 thick slice wholemeal toast
Lunch Roast pepper and feta stuffed chicken with 3 boiled baby new potatoes and Roast vegetables followed by Chocolate hazelnut mousse
Dinner Chestnut and butterbean soup and St Clement's smoothie
Snacks Antipasti skewers / Pear and 1 dsp sunflower seeds
Drinks Unlimited water, herbal teas and coffee alternatives, plus 1 glass of wine

WEEK TWO

Day 1
Breakfast Cinnamon apple porridge with 1 thin slice toasted pumpernickel style rye bread with pumpkin seed butter or peanut butter
Lunch Leek and potato soup with 2 rough oat cakes
Dinner Chilli con carne with brown basmati rice
Snacks 2 plums and 4 almonds / Tahini yoghurt
Drinks Unlimited water, herbal teas and coffee alternatives, plus 2 glasses of diluted juice

Day 2
Breakfast Low-GL granola with 2 chopped plums and milk/yoghurt
Lunch Hot smoked trout with pumpkin seed pesto and watercress open sandwich and St Clement's smoothie
Dinner Chickpea curry with brown basmati rice
Snacks 2 rough oat cakes with cottage cheese / Carrot and walnut cake
Drinks Unlimited water, herbal teas and coffee alternatives, plus 2 glasses of diluted juice

Day 3
Breakfast Low-GL granola with Rhubarb compote and yoghurt
Lunch Oriental chicken broth followed by Bresaola and artichoke hearts on rye bread
Dinner Roasted pepper rolls with goat's cheese and pine nut stuffing followed by Sun-dried tomato and black olive pesto with buckwheat pasta and a large rocket and red onion salad
Snacks Punnet of berries / Creamy tahini dip and crudités
Drinks Unlimited water, herbal teas and coffee alternatives, plus St Clement's smoothie or 1 glass of diluted juice

Day 4
Breakfast Low-carb muesli with Rhubarb compote and milk/yoghurt
Lunch Aubergine pâté with 1 wholemeal pitta bread and salad
Dinner Bangers and mash followed by Rice pudding
Snacks 2 apricots and 4 walnut halves / 1 boiled egg and 2 rough oat cakes
Drinks Unlimited water, herbal teas and coffee alternatives, plus 1 glass of diluted juice

Day 5
Breakfast 2 thin slices pumpernickel style rye bread with pumpkin seed butter or peanut butter
Lunch Greek salad followed by wholemeal pasta with Sun-dried tomato and black olive pesto
Dinner Red lentil and smoked mackerel kedgeree with steamed cauliflower followed by Pear crumble
Snacks 1 apple with 3 Brazil nuts / Greek stuffed pepper
Drinks Unlimited water, herbal teas and coffee alternatives, plus a Virgin Mary and 1 glass of diluted juice

Day 6
Breakfast Plum yoghurt crunch followed by 1 thick slice wholemeal toast or 2 thin slices toasted pumpernickel style rye bread with pumpkin seed butter or peanut butter
Lunch Avocado gazpacho followed by Cashew and sesame quinoa
Dinner Pork medallions with salsa verde, with 4 small boiled baby new potatoes and salad
Snacks Antipasti skewers / Apple and almond cake
Drinks Unlimited water, herbal teas and coffee alternatives, plus 1 glass of wine

Day 7
Breakfast Smoked salmon and chive scrambled eggs on 1 thick slice wholemeal toast
Lunch Lemon and coriander chicken en papillote with brown basmati rice and steamed green beans or salad
Dinner 55g wholemeal pasta (dry weight) with Pumpkin seed pesto and a large salad
Snacks Avocado and cream cheese dip with crudités / Tamari toasted nuts
Drinks Unlimited water, herbal teas and coffee alternatives, plus one glass of diluted fruit juice and 1 glass of wine

BREAKFASTS

Yes, the age-old cliché about breakfast being the most important meal of the day really is true, particularly for anyone trying to balance their blood sugar levels and lose weight. So we've provided plenty to tempt you here, even if you're the kind of person who can't face the thought of food first thing in the morning – or who barely has time to clean their teeth, let alone cook. The recipes cover the spectrum from super-quick and easy to more elaborate concoctions for lazy weekend mornings.

Bear in mind that you need to eat protein with carbohydrate at every meal to slow down the release of sugar. Toast and jam, for instance, are pure carbohydrate – essentially, one big shot of sugar – and thus very high GL, whereas adding protein from eggs, yoghurt or milk (including soya, nut or quinoa milk) helps to lower the GL.

Remember: aim to eat 10 Ⓖ at breakfast to lose weight, and 15 Ⓖ once you have reached the maintenance phase.

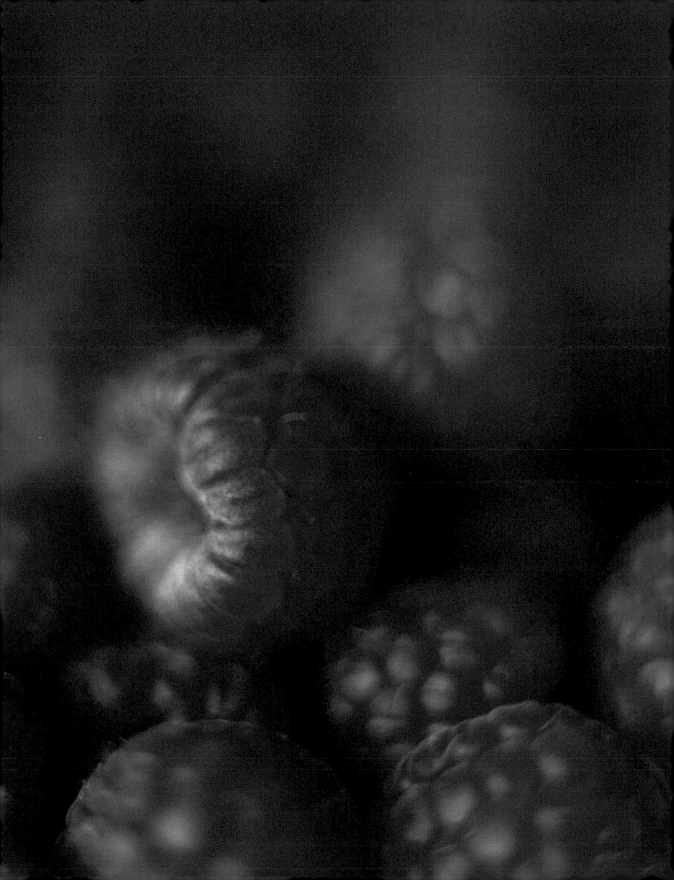

Low-GL Get Up and Go

Patrick's delicious superfood smoothie is so nutritious it will power you all the way to elevenses (and beyond!). Made from powdered wholefoods, including organic apple, flax seeds and almonds, and flovoured with natural vanilla, it is now available in a low-GL format. (See Resources, page 187, for stockists.)

(See Resources, page 187, for stockists.)

SERVES 2

2 x 30g servings Low-GL Get Up and Go
2 punnets strawberries, washed and hulled
  or 1 banana
1 pint skimmed milk, soya milk or nut milk

1 Tip all ingredients into a blender and blend till smooth.
2 Pour into 2 tall glasses and serve.

CL PER SERVING: 8.5

COOK'S NOTES
ALLERGY SUITABILITY gluten, wheat, dairy free

Toast (yes really)

We know you're more than able to make toast – we've just put this in to point out that it is primarily what you put on your toast that determines its GL rating. OK, so rye or wholemeal bread have the lowest GL of all types of bread, but you still need to have a protein-rich spread to slow down the sugar release. That means avoiding high-carb jams and marmalades in favour of the following suggestions.

SERVES 2

3 slices rye bread or 2 medium slices wholemeal bread
Peanut butter (choose a sugar-free brand), or another nut butter
  such as cashew, hazelnut or almond, or pumpkin seed butter

1 Toast the bread.
2 Spread with your chosen topping.
3 Cut the third slice of rye bread in half so that each person has 1½ slices, and serve immediately.

CL PER SERVING: 9

COOK'S NOTES
ALLERGY SUITABILITY
dairy free, go for yeast-free rye bread (available in health food stores) if you have yeast intolerance

✓ MAINTENANCE PHASE
increase to 2 slices rye bread or 1½ slices (or 1 thick slice) wholemeal bread per person (total CL = 14)

Low-carb muesli

A chewy, satisfying muesli, this is lower in carbohydrates than the classic type, as it features more nuts and seeds than grains and no dried fruit (which is very high in sugar). It is also wheat and sugar-free, unlike most of the bought varieties, but you can use a little xylitol to sweeten it if you like.

SERVES 2
100g (4oz) whole oat flakes
50g (2oz) ground almonds
2 tbsp pumpkin seeds
2 tbsp macadamia nuts, roughly chopped
2 tbsp sunflower seeds
2 tsp xylitol (optional)

Stir all the ingredients together until well mixed.

PER SERVING: 4

COOK'S NOTES
SERVING SUGGESTION (PER PERSON) serve with a tablespoon of berries per person, or fruit compote (see page 69), and a small pot of live natural yoghurt or soya yoghurt, or skimmed milk, soya milk or nut milk (total = 10)
VARIATIONS vary the nuts and seeds (pecans or hazelnuts would work well instead of the macadamia nuts)
ALLERGY SUITABILITY wheat, dairy, yeast free

MAINTENANCE PHASE double up the quantity and again serve with fruit and milk or yoghurt (total = 14)

Plum yoghurt crunch

Are you ever tempted by those fruit and yoghurt cups with a granola topping in sandwich shop and café chill cabinets? Our version tastes just as good but is wheat free and lower in saturated fat and sugar. The plums and xylitol give it sweetness, the nuts and seeds add the 'chew' factor.

SERVES 2
2 plums, de-stoned and chopped
200g (7oz) live natural yoghurt or soya yoghurt
1 tbsp linseeds
½ tbsp hazelnuts
½ tbsp macadamia nuts
½ tbsp pumpkin seeds
1 tbsp flaked almonds
1½ tsp xylitol

1 Place the chopped plums at the bottom of two short glasses.
2 Spoon the yoghurt on top.
3 Grind the linseeds in your blender or food processor, then add the hazelnuts, macadamia nuts and pumpkin seeds and continue to grind.
4 Stir the flaked almonds and xylitol into the ground mixture.
5 Sprinkle the granola mix on top of the yoghurt and serve.

PER SERVING: 4

COOK'S NOTES
SERVING SUGGESTION (PER PERSON) have 1 thin slice toasted pumpernickel style rye bread with pumpkin seed butter or peanut butter in addition to the Plum yoghurt crunch, to total 10
VARIATIONS vary the nuts and seeds. Use 1 pear, 2 apricots or a portion of fruit compote (see page 69) instead of the plums
ALLERGY SUITABILITY gluten, wheat, dariy free

MAINTENANCE PHASE
increase to 2 thin slices toasted pumpernickel style rye bread or 1 medium slice wholemeal toast in addition to the Plum yoghurt crunch (total = 15)

Low-GL granola

This easy version of the breakfast favourite tastes like a crunchy
pudding, but in fact it is extremely healthy. The oats provide soluble
fibre and low-GL wholegrain carbohydrate, while the nuts and seeds
are bursting with essential fats and minerals. The xylitol adds a little
low-GL sweetness. You may want to make this in bulk if you're pressed
for time in the mornings. For 7 days' worth of breakfasts for 2 people,
multiply all the amounts by 7, but use only 5 tbsp of the oil. Store in
the fridge to keep the nuts and seeds fresh.

SERVES 2
1 tbsp coconut oil or olive oil
1 tbsp xylitol
50g (2oz) whole oat flakes
1 tbsp flaked almonds
1 tbsp macadamia nuts, roughly chopped
1 tbsp pumpkin seeds
1 tbsp ground almonds

1 Gently melt the oil in a frying pan with the xylitol, add the oat
flakes and stir for 3 minutes or until they start to go golden and
crisp up slightly.
2 Add the flaked almonds and macadamia nuts and cook for
a further 2 minutes.
3 Remove from the heat and stir in the pumpkin seeds and
ground almonds.

Cinnamon apple porridge

When you crawl out of bed on a cold, dark winter morning, nothing
is more warming and satisfying than a steaming bowl of porridge.
We've added spice, sweetness and crunch to our version, but it's
just as quick to cook as the plain kind. Oats are full of soluble fibre
for healthy digestion and release their energy very slowly to keep
you filled up all the way through to snack time and even lunch.

SERVES 2
100g (4oz) whole porridge oats
600ml (1pt) water (or use half water and half
skimmed milk or soya or nut milk)
1 apple, cored and diced
6 tsp xylitol
1 tsp ground cinnamon plus 1/2 tsp to sprinkle on top
1 tbsp sunflower seeds or chopped nuts
   (try almonds, hazelnuts or walnuts)

1 Place the oats and water (and milk if using) in a pan along with
the apple, xylitol and teaspoon of cinnamon. Bring to the boil, then
gently simmer, stirring, until the porridge thickens and the oats
soften.
2 Pour into two bowls and sprinkle the seeds (or nuts) and the
remaining half teaspoon of cinnamon over the top before serving.

Fruit salad

An appetizing, multicoloured mix of low-GL fruits that's bursting with flavour and packed with phytonutrients and vitamins.

SERVES 2

1 kiwi fruit, peeled and thinly sliced
4 tbsp blueberries, rinsed and drained
4 handfuls of raspberries or strawberries, rinsed and drained then hulled (Tip: wash strawberries before hulling to prevent them from absorbing too much water and going soggy)

Toss all the fruit together and serve.

GL PER SERVING: 7

COOK'S NOTES
SERVING SUGGESTION (PER PERSON) serve with a small pot of live natural yoghurt or soya yoghurt (total GL = 10)
VARIATIONS vary the berries according to taste and availability
ALLERGY SUITABILITY gluten, wheat, dairy, yeast free

✓ MAINTENANCE PHASE
serve with granola (see page 68) and live natural yoghurt or soya yoghurt (total GL = 12.5), or have 1 thin slice toasted pumpernickel style rye bread or 1 medium slice wholemeal toast with pumpkin seed butter or peanut butter as well as the Fruit salad (total GL = 15)

Apple compote

This compote adds a spicy tang to Low-carb muesli or Low-GL granola and yoghurt. Apples are full of fibre and vitamins and are one of the lowest GL fruits. If you want to double or triple this recipe to have on hand for several breakfasts, it will keep in the fridge for up to 5 days, or can be frozen.

SERVES 2

1 Bramley (cooking) apple, cored and diced but unpeeled
¼ tsp ground ginger or ½ tsp ground cinnamon
1 tsp xylitol
2 tsp lemon juice

1 Place all the ingredients in a saucepan.
2 Cover and gently stew until the apples soften and start to disintegrate (this takes about 10 minutes), stirring from time to time so they do not stick to the bottom of the pan.

GL PER SERVING: 5

COOK'S NOTES
SERVING SUGGESTION (PER PERSON) serve with Low-carb muesli (see page 67) or Low-GL granola (see page 68) and milk or yoghurt (total GL = 10)
VARIATIONS use other low-GL fruits like apricots, plums, berries or pears instead of the apple
ALLERGY SUITABILITY gluten, wheat, dairy, yeast free

Rhubarb compote

Rhubarb is rich in dietary fibre and vitamin C, and deliciously tart when stewed. This fruit compote is wonderful partnered with yoghurt and Low-carb muesli, or as a pudding. If you want to double or triple this recipe to have on hand for several breakfasts, it will keep in the fridge for up to 5 days, or can be frozen.

SERVES 2

200g (7oz) trimmed and washed rhubarb, cut into chunks
Dash of water
2 tbsp xylitol

1 Place the rhubarb in a saucepan with the water and xylitol.
2 Simmer for around 10 minutes, uncovered, until soft and disintegrating.

GL PER SERVING: 5

COOK'S NOTES
SERVING SUGGESTION (PER PERSON) serve with Low-carb muesli (see page 67) and milk or a small pot of live yoghurt (total GL = 10)
ALLERGY SUITABILITY gluten, wheat, dairy, yeast free

Boiled eggs and soldiers

This one will bring back childhood memories. It's also the perfect low-GL breakfast, complete with protein and slow-releasing carbohydrate.

SERVES 2

4 medium free range eggs
3 slices rye bread or 2 medium slices wholemeal bread
A little butter (optional)

1 Bring a pan of water to a slow boil and gently place the eggs into the pan. Leave to boil gently for 4 minutes.
2 Meanwhile, toast the bread and cut into soldiers (buttered first if you can't bear the thought of dry toast, although the egg yolk contains enough fat to provide the same smooth, soft texture on its own).
3 Remove the eggs from the pan and place in egg cups alongside the toast (each person should have 1½ slices of rye bread, if you're using it).

GL PER SERVING: 9

COOK'S NOTES
ALLERGY SUITABILITY go for yeast-free rye bread (available in health food stores) if you have a yeast intolerance

MAINTENANCE PHASE
increase to 2 slices rye bread or 1½ slices (or 1 thick slice) wholemeal bread per person and use large eggs (total GL = 13)

Scrambled eggs on toast

A firm contender in the comfort food stakes. Made properly, with the eggs still a little runny, this is a fabulous dish, but if the egg is left in the pan for too long and goes dry . . . give it to the dog and start again. Life's too short for bad scrambled eggs. If you balk at unbuttered toast, rest assured that the egg yolk provides a wonderful creamy-smooth texture that stops it from being dry.

SERVES 2
4 medium free range eggs
Freshly ground black pepper
3 thin slices pumpernickel style rye bread or 2 medium slices wholemeal bread
2 tsp coconut oil or olive oil

1 Beat the eggs with the pepper.
2 Toast the bread.
3 While the bread is toasting, heat the oil in a small pan over a gentle heat and pour in the beaten eggs.
4 Slowly stir the eggs with a wooden spoon, scraping along the base of the pan as they cook to keep them moving and help stop them sticking. Remove from the heat as soon as the eggs are almost set but still a little runny/moist.
5 Serve on the toast (each person should have 1¹/2 slices rye bread, if you're using it).

PER SERVING: 9

COOK'S NOTES
SERVING SUGGESTION (PER PERSON) serve with grilled tomatoes, if liked
ALLERGY SUITABILITY wheat, dairy free

MAINTENANCE PHASE
increase to 2 thin slices toasted pumpernickel style rye bread or 1¹/2 medium slices (or 1 thick slice) wholemeal toast per person, and use large eggs (total GL = 15)

🍴 **COOK'S NOTES**
SERVING SUGGESTION (PER PERSON)
serve on 1½ thin slices toasted
pumpernickel style rye bread or
1 medium slice wholemeal toast
(total ⊕ = 10)
ALLERGY SUITABILITY gluten, wheat,
dairy, yeast free

✅ **MAINTENANCE PHASE**
spoon into a toasted pitta bread or
onto 1 thick slice wholemeal toast
with sliced tomatoes (total ⊕ = 14)

Scrambled eggs and mushrooms

Eggs are nutritional powerhouses, packed full of protein, iron, zinc
and B vitamins. They also taste delicious with onion and mushrooms,
as this wonderfully savoury dish shows.

SERVES 2
FOR THE ONION AND MUSHROOMS
1 tbsp coconut oil or olive oil
1 onion, finely chopped
200g (7oz) mushrooms, cleaned with a brush or wiped
  with kitchen towel and sliced
½ tsp dried herbes de Provence

FOR THE SCRAMBLED EGGS
4 medium eggs
Freshly ground black pepper
2 tsp coconut oil or olive oil
½ tsp Marigold Reduced Salt Vegetable Bouillon powder

1 Heat the tablespoon of oil in a pan and gently sauté the onion
until fairly soft, then add the mushrooms and dried herbs and allow
the mushrooms to soften and cook down. Set to one side and keep
warm until the eggs are ready.
2 Beat the eggs with the black pepper.
3 Heat the 2 teaspoons of oil in a small pan and stir in the
bouillon powder.
4 Pour the beaten eggs into the pan and slowly stir with a wooden
spoon, scraping along the base of the pan as they cook to keep
them moving and help stop them sticking. Remove from the heat
as soon as the eggs are almost set but still a little runny/moist.
5 Serve on top of the cooked mushrooms on toast (see serving
suggestion).

Smoked salmon and chive scrambled eggs

Perfect for breakfast in bed at the weekend – scrambled eggs with smoked salmon – and a beneficial dose of omega-3s (essential fatty acids that promote a healthy skin, heart and brain) along with it.

SERVES 2
4 medium eggs
Freshly ground black pepper
2 tsp coconut oil or olive oil
2 tsp fresh chives, chopped
75g (3oz) smoked salmon

1 Beat the eggs with the black pepper.
2 Heat the oil in a small pan over a gentle heat and pour in the beaten egg.
3 Slowly stir with a wooden spoon, scraping along the base of the pan as the eggs cook to keep them moving and help stop them from sticking. Remove from the heat as soon as the eggs are almost set but still a little runny/moist.
4 Sprinkle with chopped chives and serve immediately with the smoked salmon.

PER SERVING: 1

COOK'S NOTES
SERVING SUGGESTION (PER PERSON)
spoon into a toasted pitta pocket (total = 11) or onto 1½ thin slices toasted pumpernickel style rye bread or 1 medium slice wholemeal toast (total = 8)
VARIATIONS use dill instead of chives
ALLERGY SUITABILITY gluten, wheat, dairy free

MAINTENANCE PHASE
serve on 2 thin slices toasted pumpernickel style rye bread or 1 thick slice wholemeal toast (total = 11) and have a piece of fruit afterwards (to reach 15)

SAVOURY SNACKS & STARTERS

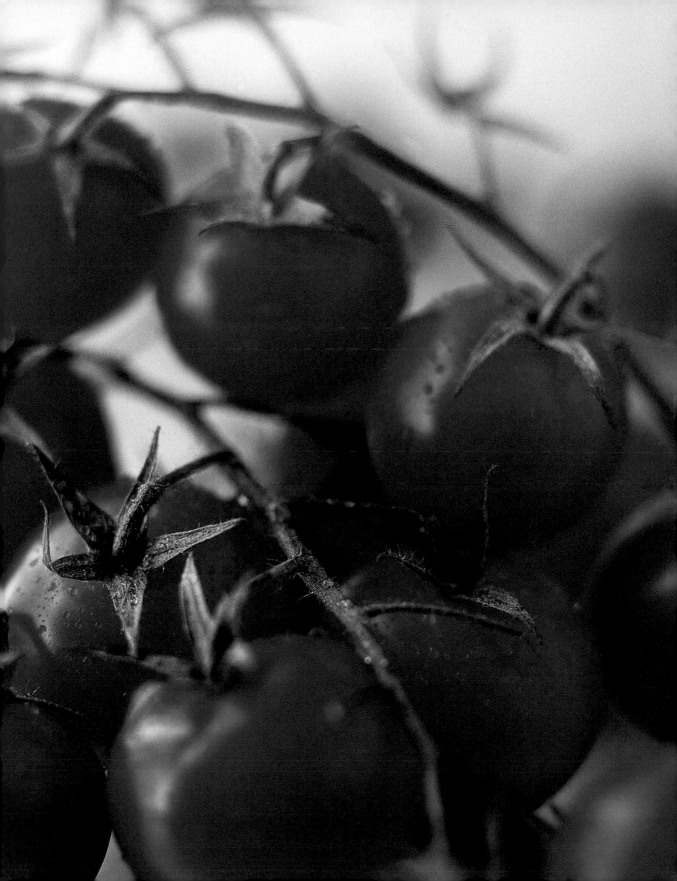

If in your former life you were always looking forward to a mid-morning packet of crisps, you won't miss it. You'll find a whole range of treats here that, in addition to having just 5 Ⓖⓛ or less, are all incredibly tasty and interesting. If you're in the weight-loss phase, they're intended as between-meal snacks. And if you have reached the maintenance phase, and need to increase your daily GL intake, you can have them as starters as well.

We've included a number of moreish dips and pâtés here that will go brilliantly either with a rough oat cake or with crudités – and raw vegetable sticks are the ideal way to add a potent antioxidant and vitamin punch to your day. Try a good handful of chopped peppers (red, orange and yellow are sweetest), and cucumber and carrot sticks. Baby spring onions, radishes, raw sugar snap peas, baby corn and cherry tomatoes are other perfect bite-sized options that simply need washing and trimming. Keep some ready prepared in an airtight container in the fridge, or take some to work with a separate container of whichever dip you fancy.

Ready-to-eat lean chicken or turkey goujons from the supermarket are another, protein-rich option with dips.

The Holford Diet is also big on fruit with seeds or nuts, or simple combinations of oat cakes with, say, cottage cheese – both useful and tasty snacks when you're pushed for time. See Part 1, page 26, for what you'll eat of these to get 5 Ⓖⓛ.

Remember: you should aim to eat 5 Ⓖⓛ for both your mid-morning and mid-afternoon snacks to lose weight, and the same once you have reached the maintenance phase.

SALAD SKEWERS

These skewer ideas are a fun, much more interesting take on the old cheese-and-pineapple-on-a stick theme. They are also very easy to eat standing up, making them the perfect drinks party canapés.

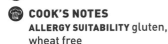

PER SERVING: 5

COOK'S NOTES
ALLERGY SUITABILITY gluten, wheat free

Greek salad skewers

Meze on a stick – refreshing and tangy.

SERVES 2
FOR THE SKEWERS
10 x 1cm square (1/2 in) cubes feta cheese
5cm long (2 in) slice of cucumber, quartered lengthways, then sliced horizontally to form small triangular slices (use 1 triangle per skewer)
3 cherry tomatoes, quartered (you'll need 10 of the pieces)
10 short slices of red onion (the same size as the cucumber)
5 Kalamata olives, pitted and halved

FOR THE DIPPING SAUCE
4 parts extra virgin oil oil to 1 part white wine vinegar
Freshly ground black pepper
Pinch of dried oregano

1 Spear the skewer ingredients onto a cocktail stick and arrange on a platter.
2 Make the dipping sauce by mixing the oil and vinegar, then seasoning to taste with pepper and oregano. Serve with the skewers in a small bowl.

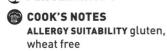

PER SERVING: 5

COOK'S NOTES
ALLERGY SUITABILITY gluten, wheat free

Antipasti skewers

These classic Mediterranean flavours complement each other perfectly.

SERVES 2
10 sun-blush tomato sections or slices of marinated roast pepper
5 black olives, pitted and halved
10 x 1cm square (1/2 in) cubes feta cheese
5 marinated artichoke hearts, halved
Oil from the antipasti jars (optional)

1 Spear the skewer ingredients onto a cocktail stick and arrange on a platter.
2 If you like, you can simply pour some of the oil from the jar of sunblush tomatoes, peppers or artichokes into a small dish for dipping.
It should have lots of flavour from any herbs or garlic in the marinade.

Tamari toasted nuts

These are irresistibly tasty, yet high in protein and minerals and low in carbohydrate and saturated fat. You can take them to work in a small sealed container, or serve as nibbles at a drinks party. You can make up to a week's worth of this snack – just store it in an airtight tin, preferably in the fridge.

SERVES 2

50g (2oz) mixed nuts and seeds (such as Brazil nuts, pecans, walnuts, almonds, pinenuts, pumpkin seeds, sesame seeds or sunflower seeds)
1 tbsp tamari (wheat-free soy sauce) or use soy sauce

1 Preheat the oven to 200C/400F/Gas mark 6.
2 Put the nuts and seeds in a baking tray, tip the tamari or soy sauce over them and shake around to coat thoroughly.
3 Roast for around 5 minutes, shaking the tray halfway through.

GL PER SERVING: 2

COOK'S NOTES
ALLERGY SUITABILITY gluten, wheat, dairy free (tamari is gluten free, but soy sauce does contain gluten)

Avocado and cream cheese dip

A winning combination of smooth, rich avocado and garlicky cream cheese, this is wonderful with a handful of crisp crudités or an oat cake, and extremely quick to whip up. Note, though, that while avocado has a very low GL, it does contain quite a lot of fat, so don't have this dip more than twice a week.

SERVES 2

1/2 ripe avocado, stone removed and the flesh scraped from the shell
75g (3oz) low-fat garlic and herb cream cheese
1/2 tsp lemon juice
Freshly ground black pepper

Mash all the ingredients together.

GL PER SERVING: 2

COOK'S NOTES
SERVING SUGGESTION (PER PERSON) use as a dip with a handful of crudités or serve with 1 rough oat cake for a 5 GL snack or starter
VARIATIONS add some finely sliced spring onions to the dip
ALLERGY SUITABILITY gluten, wheat free

Creamy tahini dip

Tahini, a paste made from pulped sesame seeds, has a strong flavour but is delicious when tempered with mild cream cheese.

SERVES 2

1 tbsp low-fat cream cheese (either plain or with garlic and herbs)
2 tsp tahini
1/2 tbsp fresh flat leaf parsley leaves, finely chopped

Thoroughly mix all the ingredients together.

GL PER SERVING: 2

COOK'S NOTES
SERVING SUGGESTION (PER PERSON) serve with 1 rough oat cake or a handful of crudités (total GL = 5)
ALLERGY SUITABILITY gluten, wheat free

Yoghurt satay dip

The nutty taste of this dip is very satisfying and goes well with raw veg. This is a simple version that's easy to prepare, light and low in fat because it's made with yoghurt.

SERVES 2
2 tbsp live natural yoghurt
2 tbsp crunchy peanut butter (choose a sugar-free brand)

Mix the ingredients together.

GL PER SERVING: 1

COOK'S NOTES
SERVING SUGGESTION (PER PERSON) serve with a handful of crudités (total **GL** = 5)
ALLERGY SUITABILITY gluten, wheat free

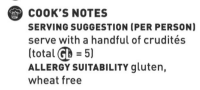

Spicy Mexican bean dip

A filling and versatile dip that is just as good with crudités as with a beefburger (see page 97) or in fajita wraps with chicken and peppers. Kidney beans are rich in phytoestrogens that help to balance hormones. You can double this recipe and store in the fridge for up to 3 days.

SERVES 2
1/4 onion, finely chopped
2 cloves of garlic, crushed
1/2 tbsp olive oil
1/4 tsp chilli powder
1 tsp lemon juice
150g (just over 5oz) kidney beans, cooked and drained
75g (3oz) cottage cheese
1 tbsp yoghurt
Low-sodium salt or sea salt
Freshly ground black pepper

1 Sauté the onion and garlic gently in the oil in a pan for around 2 minutes.
2 Add the chilli powder and cook for a further 3 minutes.
3 Cool and blend with the rest of the ingredients for a fairly smooth, creamy dip.

GL PER SERVING: 4

COOK'S NOTES
SERVING SUGGESTION (PER PERSON) serve with a handful of crudités (total **GL** = 5)
ALLERGY SUITABILITY gluten, wheat free

Red pepper and cucumber salsa

A zesty dollop of this will liven up summer meals or burgers. Raw vegetables are packed with vitamins, antioxidants and enzymes, and red onion in particular contains sulphurous amino acids that boost the body's ability to detoxify.

SERVES 2

1 medium red onion, diced
4 cherry tomatoes, cut into small chunks
1/2 red pepper, diced
1 tbsp olive oil
1 dsp fresh flat leaf parsley leaves, finely chopped
5cm (2 in) chunk of cucumber, cut lengthways into quarters
   then sliced horizontally (into triangles)
2 tsp red chilli, deseeded and finely chopped
2 tsp lemon juice
Freshly ground black pepper

Mix all the ingredients together.

PER SERVING: 2

COOK'S NOTES
SERVING SUGGESTION (PER PERSON) serve with a handful of crudités (total = 5)
VARIATIONS pep this up with more chilli if you like
ALLERGY SUITABILITY gluten, wheat, dairy, yeast free

Guacamole

Fresh chilli, garlic and spring onions give this version of the Mexican speciality a real kick. Easy to throw together in minutes.

SERVES 2

1 ripe avocado
Juice of 1/2 a lime
2 cloves of garlic, crushed
1 tbsp fresh coriander, finely chopped
4 spring onions, finely chopped
Freshly ground black pepper
1/4 mild chilli, deseeded

Mash all the ingredients together and adjust the seasoning according to taste.

PER SERVING: 1

COOK'S NOTES
SERVING SUGGESTION (PER PERSON) serve with a handful of crudités (total = 5)
VARIATIONS add some pitted and chopped black olives or some roasted peppers. Omit the chilli for a milder version
ALLERGY SUITABILITY gluten, wheat, dairy, yeast free

ⓒ COOK'S NOTES
SERVING SUGGESTION (PER PERSON)
serve with a handful of crudités
and/or chicken or turkey goujons
or cubes of smoked tofu for a 5 ⓖ
snack or starter
ALLERGY SUITABILITY gluten,
wheat free

Satay dipping sauce

A delicious version of classic satay, bursting with flavours.
It also contains lots of nutrients from the chilli, garlic, ginger
and onion – all of which aid the immune system –while the
live yoghurt provides probiotic bacteria for healthy digestion.

SERVES 2
2 tbsp live natural yoghurt
2 tbsp crunchy peanut butter (choose a sugar-free brand)
1 clove of garlic, crushed
1 tsp fresh ginger root, peeled and grated (Tip: the easiest
   way to peel root ginger is to scrape the skin off with the
   edge of a teaspoon)
1 tsp mild red chilli, deseeded and finely chopped
1 tsp lemon juice
2 tsp fresh coriander leaves, finely chopped
1 spring onion, finely sliced

Mix all the ingredients together.

Hummus and egg pâté

Egg mayo gets a makeover here, using hummus for a rich flavour.
Use ready-made hummus for this recipe, as it has a smoother,
softer consistency than home-made. You can double this recipe
and store in the fridge for up to 3 days.

ⓒ COOK'S NOTES
SERVING SUGGESTION (PER PERSON)
serve on 1 rough oat cake or as a
dip with crudités (total ⓖ = 5)
ALLERGY SUITABILITY gluten,
wheat, dairy, yeast free

SERVES 2
2 eggs, hardboiled (8 minutes), shelled
100g (4oz) hummus
1/2 tbsp fresh flat leaf parsley leaves, finely chopped
Freshly ground black pepper

1 Mash the eggs into the hummus.
2 Add the parsley and black pepper, and mix everything together.

Goat's cheese and artichoke pâté

Creamy goat's cheese complements the subtle flavour of artichoke.
This remarkable vegetable (it's actually a member of the thistle
family) is very good for the liver and can boost detoxification.

ⓒ COOK'S NOTES
SERVING SUGGESTION (PER PERSON)
serve with 1 rough oat cake or a
handful of crudités for a snack
or starter (total ⓖ = 5)
VARIATIONS add some dry black
olives (pitted and chopped) to
the pâté
ALLERGY SUITABILITY gluten,
wheat free

SERVES 2
50g (2oz) marinated artichoke hearts in oil, drained
(about 5 hearts)
50g (2oz) mild soft goat's cheese
Freshly ground black pepper

Mash all the ingredients together.

Roasted red pepper hummus

Roasted red peppers have a slightly smoky, sweet taste that adds oomph to plain hummus. They're also rich in immune-boosting antioxidants. You can double this recipe and store in the fridge for up to 3 days.

SERVES 4 AS A SNACK OR 2 AS A MAIN MEAL
1 x 410g can chickpeas, rinsed and drained
1 tbsp lemon juice
75g (3oz) or 1 large roasted red pepper, either from the deli
  or a jar or roasted yourself (see recipe on page 126)
2 cloves of garlic, crushed
1 tsp ground cumin
1 tbsp tahini
1 tbsp fresh flat leaf parsley leaves, chopped
1 tbsp extra virgin olive oil
Freshly ground black pepper

Blend all the ingredients in a food processor until smooth.

PER SERVING: 2.5 IF SERVED AS A SNACK FOR 4 PEOPLE, 5 IF SERVED AS A MAIN MEAL FOR 2

COOK'S NOTES
SERVING SUGGESTION (PER PERSON) serves 4 people with 1 rough oat cake or a handful of crudités each as a snack or starter (total GL = 5.5), or serves 2 people with 2 rough oat cakes each as a main meal (total GL =10)
VARIATIONS add some pitted and chopped black olives instead of the red pepper. For plain hummus, just omit the roasted pepper
ALLERGY SUITABILITY gluten, wheat, dairy free

MAINTENANCE PHASE
serves 2 people with 1 wholemeal pitta bread and salad each (total GL = 15)

Hummus soufflé

This recipe is utterly simple and infallible – an impressive-looking, tasty starter that is great for the maintenance phase. The beaten egg whites hold the mixture in a classic soufflé shape before you have even cooked it, avoiding the angst of waiting for a soufflé to rise. Use ready-made hummus for this recipe, as it has the soft consistency that works well in a soufflé.

SERVES 2
1 tbsp mixed pepper antipasto in oil, drained
1 tbsp fresh flat leaf parsley leaves, finely chopped
100g (4oz) hummus
2 medium egg whites

1 Preheat the oven to 190C/375F/Gas mark 5.
2 Cut the pepper antipasto into strips and place in the bottom of two ramekins.
3 Stir the parsley into the hummus.
4 Beat the egg whites until they form stiff peaks.
5 Gently fold the egg into the hummus using a metal spoon and carefully spoon into the ramekins, making a mountain shape on top like a risen soufflé (we know it's cheating, but no one else will!)
6 Bake for 15 minutes.

PER SERVING: 2

COOK'S NOTES
SERVING SUGGESTION (PER PERSON) serve with 1 rough oat cake for a 5 GL snack or serve as a delicious and unusual starter on its own for a summer dinner party
VARIATIONS use red pepper or black olive hummus if liked, available from supermarkets
ALLERGY SUITABILITY gluten, wheat, dairy free

Tip: to use up leftover egg yolks, store them in a covered container in the fridge for up to 2 days and add to scrambled eggs for breakfast (use one extra yolk per whole egg, adding them to the pan at the same time) for a rich breakfast packed with brain-boosting phospholipids.

PER SERVING: 3

COOK'S NOTES
ALLERGY SUITABILITY gluten,
wheat, dairy, yeast free

Sesame and poppy seed muffins

This recipe is pretty fabulous – a low-GL, gluten-free, dairy-free muffin with no added fat that still tastes good! You simply mix the flavourings into beaten egg whites and bake for a light, tasty treat to serve with cottage cheese, a bowl of soup or on its own. Use ready made hummus, which has a softer, lighter consistency than home made and is easier to mix with the beaten egg whites.

SERVES 2
100g (4oz) hummus
20g (just under 1oz) tahini
2 tbsp sesame seeds, toasted in a dry frying pan until golden
20g (just under 1oz) poppy seeds
2 tsp flat leaf parsley leaves, finely chopped
Freshly ground black pepper
2 medium egg whites

1 Preheat the oven to 180C/350F/Gas mark 4 and grease 2 muffin moulds.
2 Mix the hummus, tahini, sesame and poppy seeds, parsley and black pepper together.
3 Beat the egg whites until they form stiff peaks, then gently fold into the hummus mixture.
4 Spoon into the greased muffin moulds and bake for 20 minutes until fluffy and golden on top and set in the middle.

PER SERVING: 5

COOK'S NOTES
ALLERGY SUITABILITY gluten,
wheat, dairy, yeast free

Peanut butter and sunflower seed muffins

Another yummy low-carb muffin to have with a bowl of soup or on its on own as a snack.

SERVES 2
100g (4oz) crunchy peanut butter (choose one which has no added sugar)
10g (just under 1/2 oz) tahini
20g (just under 1oz) sunflower seeds, roughly chopped
2 medium eggs, separated
2 tsp fresh flat leaf parsley leaves, finely chopped
Freshly ground black pepper

1 Preheat the oven to 180C/350F/Gas mark 4 and grease 2 muffin moulds.
2 Mix the peanut butter, tahini, sunflower seeds, egg yolks, herbs and black pepper together.
3 Beat the egg whites until they form stiff peaks then gently fold into the mixture. This mixture is quite solid, so after starting with 1 tablespoon of the egg white, work slowly and carefully to mix the egg white in, while trying to preserve as much air as possible in it.
4 Spoon into the greased muffin moulds and bake for 20 minutes until fluffy and golden on top and set in the middle.

Gravadlax with quail's eggs

Gravadlax is smoked salmon cured with dill and other herbs, giving it an intense, zesty flavour. It is also packed with skin nutrients, from the omega-3 fats in the salmon to the zinc in the eggs. Here it is paired with quail's eggs for a light starter. You can hardboil the eggs ahead of time if you're serving this at a dinner party. When you're ready to shell the eggs, crack the shells lightly on your kitchen countertop, submerge the eggs in a bowl of cold water, and carefully peel them.

SERVES 2
100g (4oz) gravadlax slices
5cm (2in) chunk of cucumber, peeled and deseeded, then grated into ribbons or julienned
4 quail's eggs, hardboiled (4 minutes), peeled and halved
2 tsp lemon juice
Freshly ground black pepper

1 Arrange the gravadlax slices in a nest in the middle of each plate.
2 Place the cucumber strips within the nests.
3 Arrange the quails' egg halves in the middle of each nest.
4 Drizzle each dish with lemon juice and sprinkle with black pepper before serving.

GL PER SERVING: 1

COOK'S NOTES
SERVING SUGGESTION (PER PERSON) serve on its own as a light starter or with 1 thin slice pumpernickel style rye bread (total **GL** = 6)
VARIATIONS use smoked salmon if you can't get hold of gravadlax – or use smoked trout
ALLERGY SUITABILITY gluten, wheat, dairy free

Feta and olive roast peppers

An antipasto-style starter or snack. Peppers are a rich source of antioxidants and vitamins, while tomatoes and tomato purée are excellent sources of the powerful antioxidant lycopene.

SERVES 2
1 red pepper, quartered lengthways, with the inner core, stem and seeds removed
1/2 clove of garlic, crushed
1 tsp balsamic vinegar
1 handful of cherry tomatoes, quartered
1 tbsp Kalamata olives, pitted and halved
1 tbsp sun-dried tomato purée
50g (2oz) feta cheese
Freshly ground black pepper
1 tbsp fresh basil leaves, roughly torn

1 Preheat the oven to 200C/400F/Gas mark 6.
2 Place the peppers in a roasting tin with the cut side facing up.
3 Mix together the garlic, balsamic vinegar, cherry tomatoes, olives and sun-dried tomato purée and spoon into the cavity of each pepper quarter.
4 Bake for 25 minutes, then crumble the feta on top of each pepper quarter and sprinkle with black pepper and the basil.

GL PER SERVING: 4

COOK'S NOTES
SERVING SUGGESTION (PER PERSON) serve on their own or with green leaves as a snack or starter
VARIATIONS replace the feta with 4 anchovy fillets
ALLERGY SUITABILITY gluten, wheat free

COOK'S NOTES

SERVING SUGGESTION (PER PERSON)
serve on a bed of rocket leaves as
a 2 GF starter or have with 1 rough
oat cake as a 5 GF snack
VARIATIONS stir some pesto into
the cheese (see recipes on pages
143–4), or use cream cheese with
garlic and herbs instead of the
goat's cheese. You could also use
walnuts instead of pine nuts
ALLERGY SUITABILITY gluten,
wheat free

Roasted pepper rolls with goat's cheese and pine nut stuffing

A full-flavoured dish that can be served as a starter, or a snack at
work or at home. You can double this recipe and store in the fridge
for up to 3 days.

SERVES 2

300g (12oz) large roasted red peppers, either in halves or large pieces
  from the deli or a jar, or roasted at home (see recipe on page 126)
1 dsp lemon juice
100g (4oz) soft goat's cheese
Freshly ground black pepper
40g (around 1½oz) pine nuts
1 tbsp fresh basil leaves, finely chopped

1 If using home-roasted peppers, slit each of them up one side.
2 Open out flat, and pat dry with some kitchen towels. If using jarred
or deli peppers in oil, use the largest pieces you can find, and open
out flat.
3 Mix the lemon juice into the goat's cheese to loosen it up slightly.
4 Season well with black pepper and stir in the pine nuts and basil.
5 Divide the goat's cheese mixture between the peppers and spread
along the middle of each, lengthways.
6 Roll each pepper up to form a cylinder with the goat's cheese filling
in the centre and press between your fingers to stop it from unrolling.

GF

PER SERVING: 3

COOK'S NOTES

VARIATIONS substitute different
vegetables such as shredded pak
choi leaves for the bean sprouts,
and add more or less ginger, garlic
and chilli according to taste.
ALLERGY SUITABILITY gluten,
wheat, dairy, yeast free

Oriental chicken broth

This chicken broth is enlivened with deliciously aromatic flavours
from the Far East – ginger, garlic and chillies – and packs a powerful
antioxidant punch.

SERVES 2

1 chicken breast, trimmed of skin and fat
300ml (½ pt) water
4 tsp Marigold Reduced Salt Vegetable Bouillon powder
2cm (¾ in) fresh ginger root, peeled and finely sliced (Tip: the
  easiest way to peel ginger root is to scrape off the skin using
  the edge of a teaspoon)
2 cloves of garlic, finely sliced
1 tsp mild red chilli, deseeded and finely chopped
½ carrot, julienned
1 handful of beansprouts

1 Place the chicken breast in a small pan with the water, bouillon
powder, ginger, garlic and chilli in a small saucepan. Bring to
simmering point, cover and cook for 15 minutes.
2 Take the chicken out of the pan and shred into strips.
3 Return the chicken to the pan along with the carrot and beansprouts.
Simmer for a further 5 minutes.

Thai mushroom broth

Broths are fresh-tasting and nutrient-rich because they're cooked so fast. This savoury Thai version contains mushrooms such as shiitake which, have a smoky flavour and high nutrient value (they contain the immune-boosting substance lentinan).

SERVES 2

300ml (1/2 pt) water
2 tsp Marigold Reduced Salt Vegetable Bouillon powder
1 tsp mirin (Japanese rice cooking wine, available in the Oriental
  section of good supermarkets or food stores)
2 tsp tamari (wheat-free soy sauce) or use soy sauce
1 clove of garlic, finely sliced
1 tsp fresh root ginger, peeled and finely sliced (Tip: the
  easiest way to peel ginger root is to scrape off the skin
  using the edge of a teaspoon)
50g (2oz) mixed mushrooms (such as shiitake, oyster, chestnut),
  brushed or wiped clean with kitchen towel then sliced or torn
4 pieces baby corn, chopped into thirds
1 dsp fresh coriander leaves, chopped
4 spring onions, sliced on the diagonal

1 Place all the ingredients except the coriander and spring onions in a small pan. Simmer for 5 minutes.
2 Add the coriander and spring onions, stir and serve.

PER SERVING: 4

COOK'S NOTES

SERVING SUGGESTION (PER PERSON) serve on its own as a snack or starter
ALLERGY SUITABILITY gluten, wheat, dairy free (use tamari rather than soy sauce if you cannot eat gluten)

MAIN MEALS

When it comes to main meals, you're spoilt for choice on the Holford Diet. As you saw in Part 1, once you know the rules, you can throw together a tasty stir-fry, salad or a sandwich in a flash, and ring endless changes on any of those themes. The recipes in this section will give you a range of dishes for your repertoire, and plenty of ideas for launching out on your own. You'll find dishes to suit any occasion, from weekday suppers and packed lunches to dinner parties and barbecues.

What's more, if you're devoted to curry, burgers and bangers, you're in luck – we've devised low-GL versions so you don't have to deprive yourself. There are also superb dinner-party dishes inspired by French, Mediterranean or Oriental cooking, as well as old favourites like Moussaka and Chilli con carne. And if you are vegetarian or vegan, there are dozens of delicious meat-free and dairy-free dishes, plus variants on meat dishes (just check out the Cook's Notes for the meat recipes). Beans and lentils are an incredibly important part of the Holford Diet, as they offer a nutritional cornucopia of proteins, vitamins, fibre, complex carbohydrates and minerals. None of these low-GL delights takes more than a few minutes to whizz up, and they're full of supernutrient herbs and spices to support your immune system.

If you are having salad with a main meal, feel free to enliven them with any of the dressings we've included on pages 157–8 at the end of the vegetarian section, or go for any bought or home made ones that are relatively low in fat (opt for vinaigrettes and light dressings instead of creamy ones such as salad cream or Caesar salad dressing).

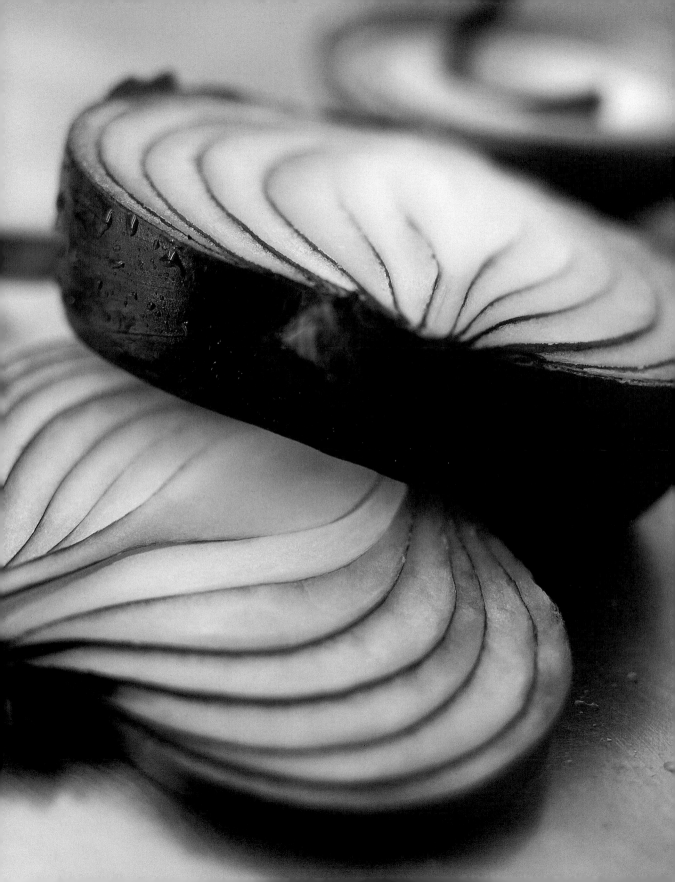

Remember: You should aim to eat 10 ⓖⓛ both at lunch and at dinner to lose weight, and 15 ⓖⓛ once you have reached the maintenance phase.

Serving suggestions, along with the total GL of a meal should you follow that serving suggestion, are included with each recipe. You can also attain your GL allowance by choosing from our appetizing accompaniments section on page 146.

Below, you'll find a table that gives you the portion sizes of the main carbohydrates. This is handy for when you've got to the point where you're balancing your own meals and want even more freedom. You can combine it with the non-starchy vegetables listed in Part 1 on page 23. For a more detailed list of the GL of foods, please consult *The Low-GL Diet Bible* and *The Holford Diet GL Counter*.

HOW BIG IS A CARBOHYDRATE SERVING?

Please note that in this table, all serving sizes are for dry weight (for example, use 45g of dried basmati rice). Cooked weights are approximately double the dried weights of rice, pasta, couscous and quinoa.

FOOD	7 ⓖⓛ SERVING (Weight-loss phase)	10 ⓖⓛ SERVING (Maintenance phase)
Brown basmati rice	45g (^{2}/$_3$ small serving)	60g (small serving)
White rice	25g (^{1}/$_3$ small serving)	30g (^{1}/$_2$ small serving)
Wholemeal pasta/spaghetti/egg pasta	40g (^{3}/$_4$ large serving)	55g (1 large serving)
White pasta/spaghetti	35g (^{1}/$_2$ serving)	45g (^{3}/$_4$ serving)
Gluten-free pasta (corn or brown rice)	20g (^{3}/$_4$ small serving)	25g (small serving)
Soba (buckwheat) noodles	20g (^{1}/$_3$ serving)	30g (^{2}/$_3$ serving)
Couscous	25g (^{1}/$_3$ medium serving)	40g (^{1}/$_2$ medium serving)
Quinoa	65g (large serving)	95g (very large serving)
Baby new potatoes (boiled)	75g (approximately 3 small)	125g (approximately 4 small)
Baked potato/sweet potato	^{1}/$_2$ small	1 small
Nairn's rough oat cakes	4	5 to 6
Rye bread (pumpernickel and sourdough varieties)	35g (1^1/$_2$ thin slices)	50g (2 thin slices)
Wholemeal bread	20g (1 medium slice or ^{3}/$_4$ thick slice)	30g (1 thick slice or 1^1/$_2$ medium slices)
Wholemeal pitta bread	25g (^{3}/$_4$ pitta bread)	30g (1 pitta bread)
Wheat tortilla wrap	40g (^{3}/$_4$ wrap)	60g (1^1/$_2$ wraps)

MEAT

Meat is a prime source of protein, and is very versatile. You may notice that we feature more recipes using lean poultry and fish than red meat, as it is important to limit your intake of saturated fat.

Venison is a leaner alternative to beef, lamb and pork, and is now available in many supermarkets and better butchers, so we have included some good recipes here among a varied and delicious array. Where possible, buy organic or at least free-range meat to limit your consumption of toxic nasties.

Chicken satay wrap

The spicy flavours of satay sauce make an interesting addition
to a classic chicken wrap.

SERVES 2
2 small wraps (widely available in supermarkets)
2 portions of Satay dipping sauce (see page 82)
1 cooked chicken breast, skinned and cut into strips
Good handful of iceburg lettuce
8 thin slices of cucumber

1 Heat the wraps in a dry frying pan for a couple of minutes on
each side to lightly toast them.
2 Spread the Satay dipping sauce in the middle of each wrap and
place the chicken and salad on top.
3 Fold both sides of the wrap into the middle and tuck the end
up to secure the parcel.

Chicken with aubergine and peppers

In this warming dish the vegetables and tomato passata cook down
into a rich stew. The onions and garlic add plenty of flavour and
antioxidants. You can double this recipe and freeze the remainder,
or store in the fridge for up to 3 days.

SERVES 2
1 tbsp coconut oil or olive oil
2 chicken breasts, trimmed of fat and skin and sliced
  into strips
2 cloves of garlic, crushed
2 tsp ground cumin
2 large red onions, diced
1 red pepper, diced
1/2 medium aubergine, diced
1 tsp Marigold Reduced Salt Vegetable Bouillon powder
200g (7oz) tomato passata
Freshly ground black pepper
1 tbsp fresh basil leaves, roughly torn

1 Heat the oil in a frying pan and sear the chicken strips on all sides,
then remove from the pan and set to one side.
2 Add the garlic and cumin to the pan and fry for 30 seconds or so before
adding the onions and pepper. Cook this mixture for about a minute.
3 Next tip in the aubergine and sauté gently for a few minutes until
all the vegetables soften (this will take about 5 minutes).
4 Return the chicken to the pan along with the bouillon powder
and passata, and simmer for 10 to 15 minutes until the meat is
properly cooked.
5 Season with black pepper and sprinkle with basil before serving.

Chicken curry

Curry nights are not out of bounds on the Holford Diet. Coconut milk and immune-boosting spices make this delicious version creamy yet piquant. You can double this recipe and freeze the remainder, or store in the fridge for up to 3 days.

SERVES 2

1 tbsp coconut oil or olive oil
2 chicken breasts, trimmed of skin and fat and sliced into strips
1 tsp ground cumin
1/2 tsp turmeric
4 cloves garlic, crushed
1 mild red chilli, deseeded and finely chopped
2 onions, chopped
2 tsp Marigold Reduced Salt Vegetable Bouillon powder dissolved in 210ml (7fl. oz) water
210ml (7fl. oz) coconut milk

1 Heat the oil in a frying pan or wok and sear the chicken strips on both sides then remove from the pan and set to one side.
2 Fry the cumin and turmeric in the pan for a few seconds before adding the garlic and chilli and sautéing for 30 seconds.
3 Add the onion and fry to soften them.
4 Pour the bouillon liquid into the pan with the coconut milk, return the meat to the pan and simmer until the chicken is cooked – about 20 to 30 minutes.

PER SERVING: 3

COOK'S NOTES
SERVING SUGGESTION (PER PERSON) serve with 45g brown basmati rice (dry weight) (total Gᴸ = 10)
VARIATIONS add 25g crunchy peanut butter (with no added sugar) and 25g tomato passata along with the coconut milk, to make a delicious satay chicken curry – in which case, use only one chicken breast between two people
ALLERGY SUITABILITY gluten, wheat, dairy, yeast free

MAINTENANCE PHASE
increase the brown basmati rice to 60g (dry weight) (total Gᴸ = 13)

Roast pepper and feta stuffed chicken

The pesto used as stuffing in this recipe has a glorious colour and a rich flavour, melting beautifully in the cooked chicken.

SERVES 2

2 chicken breasts, trimmed of skin and fat
1 portion of Feta and roast pepper pesto (see page 143)
1 tbsp olive oil

1 Preheat the oven to 190C/375F/Gas mark 5.
2 Make a slit along the length of each chicken breast with a small, sharp knife and insert a finger in the slit to make a pocket in the breast.
3 Stuff the breasts with the pesto and place on a baking tray. Drizzle the oil over the breasts and bake for 25 minutes (or until the chicken is cooked).

PER SERVING: 1

COOK'S NOTES
SERVING SUGGESTION (PER PERSON) serve with Sweet potato wedges (see page 152) and roasted courgettes (total Gᴸ = 10)
VARIATIONS stuff with any of the other pesto recipes on pages 142–4
ALLERGY SUITABILITY gluten, wheat free

MAINTENANCE PHASE
serve with Roasted vegetables (see page 150) and 4 small boiled baby new potatoes (total Gᴸ = 16)

Sesame chicken and soba noodle steam-fry

Soba noodles are made from buckwheat, a gluten-free seed with an earthy, grain-like taste. They cook quickly in 4 to 6 minutes and make an interesting change from wheat noodles or rice.

SERVES 2
2 tsp coconut oil or olive oil
2 cloves of garlic, crushed
2 tsp chopped fresh root ginger (Tip: the easiest way to peel root ginger is to scrape away the skin with the edge of a teaspoon)
2 chicken breasts, trimmed of skin and fat and sliced into strips
4 handfuls of chopped mixed vegetables (try peppers, carrots, baby corn, mangetout, broccoli)
2 tsp Marigold Reduced Salt Vegetable Bouillon powder
2 tbsp water
100g (4oz) soba noodles
2 tsp sesame oil

1 Heat the oil in a wok and stir-fry the garlic, ginger and chicken over a moderate heat for 2 minutes or so until the meat is coloured on all sides.
2 Add the vegetables, bouillon powder and water to the wok and place the lid on immediately. Cook for 5 to 7 minutes to let the vegetables soften and the meat finish cooking, checking halfway through to make sure the water hasn't evaporated. If it has, add another tablespoon or so and replace the lid.
3 Meanwhile, cook the noodles. Put in a pan of boiling water, cover and boil for 4 to 6 minutes, then drain and rinse under cold water. Take care not to overcook them.
4 Tip the noodles into the wok, add the sesame oil, stir all the ingredients together and serve.

PER SERVING: 10

COOK'S NOTES
ALLERGY SUITABILITY gluten, wheat, dairy, yeast free (make you sure you choose 100 per cent buckwheat soba noodles if you are gluten intolerant – some of them also contain wheat)

MAINTENANCE PHASE
serve with a 5 GL starter or pudding (total GL = 15)

Teriyaki chicken

Teriyaki is a savoury Japanese sauce with great depth of flavour that transforms chicken, fish or tofu. Our version uses the naturally low-carbohydrate, low-calorie sweetener xylitol instead of sugar, and tamari, a wheat-free version of soy sauce.

SERVES 2
2 chicken breasts, trimmed of fat and skin and cut into strips
2 portions of Teriyaki sauce (see page 157)
1 tbsp coconut oil or olive oil

1 If you have time, marinate the chicken in the Teriyaki sauce for around 30 minutes in the fridge. If you're starving and impatient, simply toss the meat in the sauce.
2 Heat the oil in a large frying pan and place the chicken (without the marinade liquid if there is any remaining) in the pan. Stir-fry on a low heat for around 5 minutes, turning the strips over halfway through to let the meat start to turn golden on all sides, and serve.

PER SERVING: 1

COOK'S NOTES
SERVING SUGGESTION (PER PERSON) serve with 45g brown basmati rice (dry weight) and steam-fried vegetables (total GL = 10)
ALLERGY SUITABILITY gluten, wheat, dairy free

MAINTENANCE PHASE
increase the brown basmati rice to 60g (dry weight) and serve with lots of steam-fried or stir-fried vegetables (total GL = 14)

Lemon and coriander chicken en papillote

This recipe started as a complete experiment but was so successful that it appears here. Cooking en papillote (essentially, steaming the food in its own juices in a parcel of baking parchment) is a very gentle way of cooking and preserves the flavours. And as everything cooks together in the parcel, there is no juggling of pans or need to get timings right.

SERVES 2

2 chicken breasts, trimmed of fat and skin
2 handfuls of bean sprouts
2 handfuls of baby corn (about 8)
2 tsp mild red chilli, deseeded and finely chopped
2 cloves of garlic, crushed
2 tsp fresh root ginger, peeled and finely chopped (Tip: the easiest way to peel ginger is to use the edge of a teaspoon to scrape the skin off)
1 tbsp coriander, finely chopped
2 tbsp olive oil
1 tbsp tamari (wheat free soy sauce, or use soy sauce)
2 tsp lemon juice

1 Preheat the oven to 190C/375F/Gas mark 5.
2 Cut a large square of baking paper (big enough to fold in half, diagonally, over the chicken breasts and seal up the edges to make a triangular-shaped parcel) and place on a baking sheet.
3 Mix the chicken, bean sprouts and baby corn together with all the rest of the ingredients.
4 Place in the middle of the square of paper and fold in half on the diagonal, point to point, to make a triangle. Starting at on end, make small overlapping folds around the edge, working your way round to seal the parcel (you can secure the last fold with a paperclip if you like, or just fold it underneath).
5 Bake for 25 minutes. Open the parcel with care, as you'll want to retain the cooking liquid – this is a delicious sauce or dressing on noodles or rice – and dish out onto two plates.

PER SERVING: 2

COOK'S NOTES
SERVING SUGGESTION (PER PERSON) serve with 45g brown basmati rice (dry weight) (total GL = 9)
VARIATIONS use mangetout or sugarsnap peas instead of the baby corn or bean sprouts
ALLERGY SUITABILITY gluten, wheat, dairy free

MAINTENANCE PHASE increase the brown basmati rice to 65g (dry weight) (total GL = 14)

Chicken with cherry tomatoes and crème fraîche

A McDonald Joyce family supper and dinner party staple that we are sure will become a firm favourite with you as well. It's exceptionally easy, yet very impressive. The tomatoes cook down to release their juice, which, combined with the crème fraîche, makes a wonderfully creamy sauce. You can double this recipe and store in the fridge for up to 3 days.

SERVES 2
2 tbsp olive oil
2 chicken breasts, trimmed of fat and skin
225g (8oz) cherry tomatoes
1½ tbsp low-fat crème fraîche
1 tbsp basil leaves, chopped or roughly torn
Freshly ground black pepper

1 Preheat the oven to 200C/400F/Gas mark 6.
2 Pour the oil into a shallow ovenproof dish (one that can also go on the hob) and add the chicken breasts, turning to coat in the oil.
3 Place the whole cherry tomatoes around the chicken in the dish and cook for around 50 to 60 minutes or until the chicken is done, basting occasionally.
4 Place the dish on the hob and add the crème fraîche. Heat gently until it starts to bubble, then simmer for a moment until the sauce thickens.
5 Stir in the basil and season with black pepper.

PER SERVING: 4

COOK'S NOTES
SERVING SUGGESTION (PER PERSON)
serve with 3 small boiled baby new potatoes or half a baked potato and a green salad (total = 11)
ALLERGY SUITABILITY
gluten, wheat free

MAINTENANCE PHASE
increase to 4 small boiled baby new potatoes or 1 small baked potato and a large green salad (total = 15)

Spiced turkey burgers

The alternative burger. Not only is turkey mince much leaner than pork, beef or lamb, but the garlic, chilli and other ingredients give these burgers a spicy kick.

SERVES 2 (MAKING 2 BURGERS EACH)
250g (9oz) turkey mince
1 egg yolk, beaten
4 spring onions, finely chopped
1 mild red chilli, deseeded and with the white pith removed
2 cloves of garlic, crushed
½ tsp ground cumin
½ tsp ground coriander
Freshly ground black pepper

1 Mix the turkey mince with the rest of the ingredients and leave to sit in the fridge to marinate for at least an hour.
2 Shape into burgers and grill under a medium heat for 10 minutes, then turn and grill for a further 7 minutes.

PER SERVING: 1

COOK'S NOTES
SERVING SUGGESTION (PER PERSON)
serve with Sweet potato wedges (see page 152) and Red pepper and cucumber salsa (see page 81) or Guacamole (see page 81) and lettuce (total = 11)
ALLERGY SUITABILITY
gluten, wheat, dairy, yeast free

MAINTENANCE PHASE
serve in 1 toasted wholemeal pitta bread with Red pepper and cucumber salsa (see page 81) or Guacamole (see page 81) and lettuce (total = 13)

Bresaola and artichoke hearts on rye

Here artichoke takes the place of butter, as it's wonderfully soft and squashes easily for spreading. Wholegrain rye bread and bresaola – lean, air-dried beef from Italy – make this an unusual and delicious open sandwich.

SERVES 2

2 slices of thin pumpernickel style rye bread (check the packet to make sure it is wheat free, as some brands sneak wheat in)
4 marinated artichoke hearts, drained
8 wafer-thin slices of bresaola
Freshly ground black pepper

1 Toast the rye bread if you like.
2 Mash the artichoke hearts with a fork, then spread them on the rye bread.
3 Lay the slices of bresaola on top and season with black pepper.

GL PER SERVING: 7

COOK'S NOTES
SERVING SUGGESTION (PER PERSON) have a 3 GL starter (such as Oriental chicken broth – see page 86) or pudding (like Apricot amaretti biscuits – see page 175) to make this a 10 GL main meal
VARIATIONS use thinly sliced cooked chicken or turkey from the deli or leftovers in place of the bresaola
ALLERGY SUITABILITY wheat, dairy free

✓ **MAINTENANCE PHASE**
double up the quantities per serving to have 2 sandwiches each for a 14 GL main meal

Nick's beefburgers

These burgers are delicious served with Spicy Mexican bean dip (see page 80). They're perfect for barbecues , as you can make them in advance and chill until you are ready to cook them.

SERVES 2

200g (7oz) extra lean beef mince
1 tbsp tamari (wheat-free soy sauce) or use soy sauce
1 tsp Worcestershire sauce
1 tbsp finely chopped fresh coriander
1/4 red onion, finely chopped
1/2 egg, beaten
1/2 tsp sea salt
1/2 tsp black pepper

1 Mix all ingredients apart from the mince together, then add to the mince and knead the mixture thoroughly.
2 Divide into 4 patties and flatten each into burgers.
3 Place on a plate and cover, then put in the fridge to firm up for approximately 10 minutes or until required.
4 Grill under a medium heat for approximately 7 minutes per side (or to taste).

GL PER SERVING: 1

COOK'S NOTES
SERVING SUGGESTION (PER PERSON) serve with 1/2 a wholemeal pitta bread and Spicy Mexican bean dip (see page 80) with lettuce (total GL = 10)
ALLERGY SUITABILITY dairy free

✓ **MAINTENANCE PHASE**
increase to 1 wholemeal pitta bread and serve with the Spicy Mexican bean dip and lettuce (total GL = 15)

PER SERVING: 11

COOK'S NOTES

VARIATIONS serve the sausages with Sweet potato and carrot mash instead of Cannellini bean mash, and omit the Giant baked beans (total GL = 12), or serve with 1 portion of Giant baked beans per person and no Cannellini bean mash (total GL = 10)

ALLERGY SUITABILITY (gluten, wheat), dairy free (check the sausages for gluten and wheat)

MAINTENANCE PHASE
increase the Giant baked beans to 1 portion per person (total GL = 15)

Bangers and mash

There's nothing quite like a plate of good-quality sausages and mash. As potatoes are very high GL, we've come up with a thick, comforting Cannellini bean mash instead.

SERVES 2

4 good-quality, lean sausages (venison are the leanest – look out for them at farmers' markets or buy direct from the producer via mail order or the Internet)
2 portions of Cannellini bean mash (see page 150)
1 portion of Giant baked beans (to be shared between two people – see page 153)

1 Cook the sausages according to the pack instructions (grill or oven cook rather than frying to cut down on the fat content).
2 Meanwhile, make the Cannellini bean mash and Giant baked beans. Serve with the sausages.

PER SERVING: 5

COOK'S NOTES

SERVING SUGGESTION (PER PERSON) serve with a green leaf, tomato and basil salad and have a 5 GL starter or pudding to total 10 GL

ALLERGY SUITABILITY gluten, wheat, dairy, yeast free

MAINTENANCE PHASE
serve with 4 small boiled baby new potatoes or 1 small baked potato and salad leaves (and no pudding or starter) (total GL = 15)

Tip: to use up leftover egg yolks, store them in a covered container in the fridge for up to 2 days and add to scrambled eggs for breakfast (use one extra yolk per whole egg, adding them to the pan at the same time) for a rich breakfast packed with brain-boosting phospholipids.

Moussaka

The traditional Greek dish gets a low-fat, low-GL makeover here, as it uses lean beef rather than lamb and a light soufflé crust rather than the classic cheese sauce.

SERVES 2

2 portions of Bolognese sauce (from the Spaghetti Bolognese recipe on page 100 – simply omit the spaghetti)
1 tbsp coconut oil or olive oil
1 small aubergine, sliced lengthways into about 6 slices
2 medium egg whites
100g (4oz) ready-made hummus

1 Preheat the oven to 190C/375F/Gas mark 5.
2 Make the Bolognese sauce as per the recipe instructions.
3 While that is cooking, heat the oil in a large frying pan and gently fry the aubergine slices for around 2 minutes on each side until they turn golden and soften. Remove from the pan and set to one side to cool.
4 Beat the egg whites until they form stiff peaks. Using a metal spoon to prevent air escaping from the beaten egg, take one spoonful and fold gently into the hummus. Gradually fold the rest of the egg white into the hummus, taking care not to get rid of the air.
5 Place the Bolognese sauce into a small ovenproof dish, then arrange the aubergine slices on top (try to cover the whole mixture). Carefully spoon the soufflé mixture on top and bake for 15 minutes, until the topping is golden and slightly stiff to the touch.

Chilli con carne

This hot and spicy classic is better made in advance to allow the flavours to develop and mingle. So if you're organized, you can cool it, pop it into the fridge and have it the next evening as an easy supper – just heat through and serve. This version uses more vegetables than standard recipes to optimize the nutrient content. Quantities are doubled here so you can serve the other half the day after, or freeze it.

SERVES 4

450g (1lb) lean organic beef mince
2 tsp coconut oil or olive oil
1 onion, diced
2 cloves of garlic, crushed
1 red pepper, diced
2 tsp ground cumin
1 tsp chilli powder
1–2 tsp crushed chilli flakes (according to taste)
250g (9oz) mushrooms, cleaned with a brush or wiped with
   kitchen towel and sliced
1 x 400g can chopped tomatoes
3 tbsp tomato purée
4 tsp Marigold Reduced Salt Vegetable Bouillon powder
1 x 410g can kidney beans, rinsed and drained
Freshly ground black pepper

1 Cook the mince in a large frying pan until it starts to turn grey/brown, scooping off any fat that appears with a teaspoon. Set aside.
2 Heat the oil in a separate pan and fry the onion, garlic and pepper for a couple of minutes.
3 Add the cumin, chilli powder and chilli flakes to the pan with the vegetables and cook for 10 minutes or so.
4 Add the mushrooms to the pan and cook for a further 5 minutes until soft.
5 Add the mince together with the chopped tomatoes, tomato purée, bouillon powder and kidney beans. Cover and simmer for 10 to 15 minutes, until the vegetables are soft and the flavours have mingled. Season with black pepper.

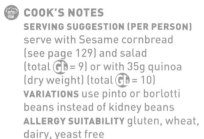

PER SERVING: 7

COOK'S NOTES
SERVING SUGGESTION (PER PERSON)
serve with Sesame cornbread (see page 129) and salad (total ⓖ = 9) or with 35g quinoa (dry weight) (total ⓖ = 10)
VARIATIONS use pinto or borlotti beans instead of kidney beans
ALLERGY SUITABILITY gluten, wheat, dairy, yeast free

MAINTENANCE PHASE
serve with 45g brown basmati rice (dry weight) and a green salad (total ⓖ = 15)

Spaghetti Bolognese

A really filling but low-GL version of spag bol, made with lean organic beef and bags of vegetables to lower the saturated fat content and provide more fibre. Quantities are doubled here so you can serve the other half next day, or freeze it.

SERVES 4
450g (1lb) lean organic beef mince
2 tsp coconut oil or olive oil
1 onion, diced
2 cloves of garlic, crushed
1 red pepper, diced
200g (7oz) mushrooms, cleaned with a brush or wiped with
   kitchen towel and sliced
1 x 400g can chopped tomatoes
3 tbsp tomato purée
3 tsp Marigold Reduced Salt Vegetable Bouillon powder
1/2–1 tsp dried oregano (according to taste)
Freshly ground black pepper

Plus 80g (3 1/4 oz) wholemeal spaghetti

1 Cook the mince in a large frying pan until it starts to turn grey/ brown, scooping off any fat that appears with a teaspoon. Set aside.
2 Heat the oil in a separate pan and fry the onion and garlic for a couple of minutes.
3 Add the diced pepper and place the lid on to sweat for 3 minutes.
4 Add the mushrooms and replace the lid to sweat for a further 3 minutes.
5 Transfer the vegetables to a large stockpot or pan and add the mince together with the chopped tomatoes, tomato purée, bouillon powder and oregano. Cover and simmer for 5 to10 minutes, until the vegetables are soft. Season with black pepper.
6 While you are waiting for the Bolognese sauce to finish cooking, cook the spaghetti according to the pack instructions. Drain and serve with the sauce.

Venison sausage and mixed pepper casserole

Venison has a rich flavour, perfectly complemented in this recipe by the sweet peppers and red onion. It's also a very lean meat and an excellent source of protein. Look for good-quality venison sausages at your local farmers' market or from organic suppliers – the ones from supermarkets are often full of additives and fillers and don't taste the same at all. You can double this recipe and freeze the remainder, or store in the fridge for up to 3 days.

SERVES 2

3 peppers (mixed colours), deseeded and sliced
1 red onion, sliced
3 tbsp tomato purée
1 tsp Marigold Reduced Salt Vegetable Bouillon powder
4 venison sausages
Freshly ground black pepper

1 Preheat the oven to 190C/375F/Gas mark 5.
2 Place the chopped peppers and onion into a shallow casserole dish and stir in the tomato purée and bouillon powder.
3 Bake for 10 minutes, then stir and place the sausages on top. Return to the oven for a further 30 to 40 minutes or until the sausages are cooked, turning halfway through.
4 Season generously with black pepper.

ⓖ PER SERVING: 4

☺ COOK'S NOTES

SERVING SUGGESTION (PER PERSON) serve with ½ a baked potato or sweet potato or 3 small boiled baby new potatoes (total ⓖ = 11)
VARIATIONS use lean, organic beef or pork sausages instead of venison
ALLERGY SUITABILITY (gluten, wheat), dairy free (as long as the sausages are gluten free)

✔ MAINTENANCE PHASE
serve with 1 small baked potato or sweet potato, or 4 small boiled baby new potatoes (total ⓖ = 14), or Roast butternut squash with shallots (see page 153) – in which case you can have a 3 ⓖ drink or pudding (to total 15 ⓖ)

COOK'S NOTES

SERVING SUGGESTION (PER PERSON)
serve on its own as a light starter
or with 3 small boiled baby new
potatoes for a main meal (total
GI = 9)
ALLERGY SUITABILITY gluten,
wheat free

✓ **MAINTENANCE PHASE**
serve with 5 small new potatoes
(total GI = 14)

Smoked venison, Parmesan and mushroom salad

The combination of smoky meat, peppery rocket and salty Parmesan
in this salad really works. This can be done in a flash and it's an
impressive dish that is well worth trying.

SERVES 2

1 tsp coconut oil or olive oil
150g (just over 5oz) mushrooms, cleaned with a brush or wiped
    with kitchen towel and sliced into thick chunks
1/2 tsp Marigold Reduced Salt Vegetable Bouillon powder
50g (2oz) watercress
50g (2oz) rocket
50g (2oz) Parmesan shavings
100g (4oz) smoked venison slices (available from good delis and
    supermarkets, or mail order direct from suppliers)
Drizzle of balsamic vinegar
Freshly ground black pepper

1 Heat the oil in a frying pan and add the mushrooms and bouillon
powder, sautéing for a few minutes to let the mushrooms cook.
Set aside to cool slightly.
2 Mix the watercress and rocket together and place on 2 plates.
3 Add the Parmesan shavings, mushrooms and venison slices to
each plate and drizzle with a little balsamic vinegar. Season with
pepper and serve.

Pork medallions with watercress salsa verde

A great low-fat alternative to chicken or fish, these grilled pork medallions are paired with sharp, herby salsa verde for a kick of fresh flavour and phytonutrients. This recipe makes enough salsa verde for 4 servings, so you can serve it the next day with fish, or mixed with beans or potatoes to make a delicious salad (it keeps for up to 5 days in the fridge).

SERVES 2
2 lean trimmed pork medallions

FOR THE WATERCRESS SALSA VERDE
1 clove of garlic, crushed
4 anchovy fillets, drained
1 tbsp capers, rinsed to remove the vinegar and drained
2 tbsp fresh flat leaf parsley leaves
1 tbsp fresh basil leaves
Good handful of watercress, roughly chopped
Freshly ground black pepper
2 tbsp extra virgin olive oil
1 tbsp lemon juice

1 Preheat the grill to a moderate heat and grill the medallions for 15 minutes (or until properly cooked), turning halfway.
2 Meanwhile, make the salsa verde. Place the salsa ingredients in a mini food processor and blitz until the sauce is well combined. (Or you can do this by hand, chopping everything very finely and mixing it all together with the oil and lemon juice.)
3 Serve a dollop of the salsa on top of each medallion.

PER SERVING: 3

COOK'S NOTES
SERVING SUGGESTION (PER PERSON) serve with 3 small boiled baby new potatoes and a green salad (total = 10)
VARIATIONS the salsa goes well with beef, tuna or trout, or simply stirred through mixed pulses or over potatoes
ALLERGY SUITABILITY gluten, wheat, dairy free (buy capers stored in sea salt rather than vinegar if you cannot eat yeast)

MAINTENANCE PHASE
increase to 4 baby new potatoes and serve with a tomato and red onion salad as well as the green leaves (total = 14)

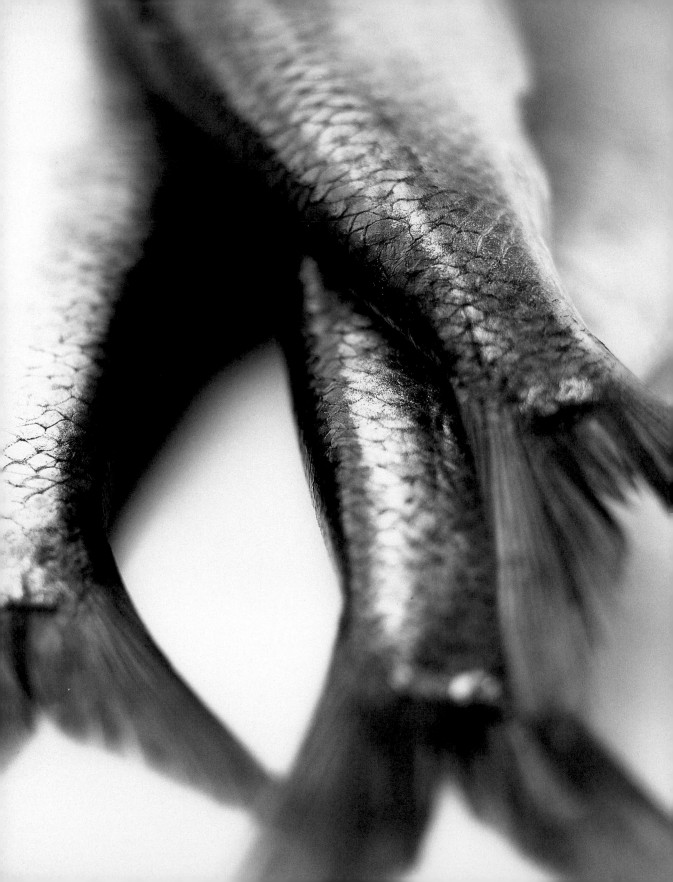

FISH

A catch indeed, fish is a superfood full of high-quality protein and ranging in flavour from the delicate to the robust. It also cooks fast, and is hugely versatile. As you'll see in this section, it takes kindly to all kinds of treatments, from smooth and creamy sauces to the classic flavours of herbs, lemon and garlic.

You'll note that we have tended to concentrate on oily coldwater fish such as salmon, trout and mackerel. Not only are they all delicious; these fish are also all rich in omega-3s, which as we've seen are essential for many aspects of health, from brainpower to hormonal balance. Note, however, that tuna – a large carnivorous fish high up the food chain – contains relatively high levels of mercury and so shouldn't be eaten more than once a month.

⊕ **COOK'S NOTES**
SERVING SUGGESTION (PER PERSON)
serve with Cannellini bean mash
(see page 150) and a green salad
(total ⊕ = 10)
VARIATIONS replace the haddock
with a boned salmon fillet (or
another white fish)
ALLERGY SUITABILITY gluten, wheat,
dairy free

✓ **MAINTENANCE PHASE**
serve with a small baked potato or 4
small boiled baby new potatoes and
a green salad (total ⊕ = 15)

> Tip: to use up leftover egg yolks,
> store them in a covered container in
> the fridge for up to 2 days and add to
> scrambled eggs for breakfast (use
> one extra yolk per whole egg, adding
> them to the pan at the same time)
> for a rich breakfast packed with
> brain-boosting phospholipids.

Seafood soufflé pie

With its soufflé topping – a wonderfully light alternative to
the usual mashed potatoes – and the addition of fresh seafood,
this is a delicious and unusual pie. Ideal for a summer supper
with friends.

SERVES 2
1 medium undyed smoked haddock fillet
300ml (1/2 pt) skimmed milk, soya milk or nut milk
300ml (1/2 pt) water
125g (just under 5oz) fresh cooked seafood selection, drained
    (such as king prawns, mussels and squid rings) from the
    supermarket chiller cabinet
2 tbsp cornflour
2 tbsp tahini
2 tsp Marigold Reduced Salt Vegetable Bouillon powder
Freshly ground black pepper
2 medium egg whites
1 tbsp fresh flat leaf parsley, finely chopped

1 Preheat the oven to 190C/375F/Gas mark 5.
2 Place the haddock in a deep frying pan and cover with the milk
and water. Bring to the boil, then simmer for 7 to 8 minutes until
the fish is cooked (the flesh should flake easily when pressed).
3 Remove the fish from the pan, reserving the poaching liquid.
Peel off the skin and flake into bite-sized chunks, then place
these in an ovenproof dish along with the drained seafood.
4 To make the sauce, pour the reserved poaching liquid into
a jug and mix in the cornflour, tahini and bouillon powder until
smooth. Pour into a smaller saucepan and gently heat, stirring
constantly, until the mixture forms a smooth, thick sauce.
Season with black pepper.
5 Pour half of the sauce over the fish and seafood in the dish
and place the other half in a large mixing bowl.
6 Beat the egg whites until they form stiff peaks.
7 Using a metal spoon, gently fold the egg whites into the
reserved sauce in the mixing bowl along with the parsley.
Then carefully spoon this soufflé mixture on top of the fish
in the ovenproof dish.
8 Bake in the middle of the oven for 15 minutes or until the
soufflé topping is light golden on top and slightly firm to
the touch.

Poached haddock with cannellini bean mash

A kind of deconstructed fish pie, with low-GL, high-fibre beans instead of mashed potatoes, and smoked haddock. Fast, easy and very tasty.

SERVES 2

2 medium undyed smoked haddock fillets
300ml (1/2 pt) skimmed milk, soya milk or nut milk
  (or enough to cover the fish in the pan to poach)
300ml (1/2 pt) water
2 portions Cannellini bean mash (see page 150)

1 Poach the haddock by placing the fillets in a deep frying pan and covering them with the milk and water. Bring to the boil, then simmer gently for 7 to 8 minutes until cooked (the flesh should flake easily when pressed).
2 Meanwhile, make the bean mash according to the recipe, and serve with the fish.

PER SERVING: 8

COOK'S NOTES
SERVING SUGGESTION (PER PERSON) serve with steamed broccoli (total GL = 10)
ALLERGY SUITABILITY gluten, wheat, dairy free

MAINTENANCE PHASE
serve with Flageolet beans in white sauce (see page 154) instead of Cannellini bean mash, and steamed broccoli (total GL = 13)

Creamy salmon with leeks

Real comfort food, with a wonderfully creamy sauce. This dish also packs a substantial nutritional punch from the omega-3s, green veg, and fibre-rich butterbeans.

SERVES 2

2 tsp coconut oil or olive oil
2 courgettes, thinly sliced horizontally
4 leeks, thinly sliced horizontally
75g (3oz) low fat cream cheese
210ml (7fl oz) skimmed milk, soya milk or nut milk
2 tbsp cornflour
1 x 410g can butterbeans, rinsed and drained
100g (4oz) smoked salmon, torn into strips
4 spring onions, finely sliced diagonally
2 tsp dill, chopped

1 Heat the oil in a large frying pan or wok and sauté the courgettes and leeks until they start to soften and colour.
2 Add the cream cheese and half the milk and stir while the cream cheese melts.
3 Mix the cornflour with the rest of the milk to form a smooth liquid and add to the pan, stirring constantly to avoid any lumps as the sauce thickens.
4 Tip in the drained butterbeans, smoked salmon, spring onions and dill and heat through.

PER SERVING: 8

COOK'S NOTES
SERVING SUGGESTION (PER PERSON) serve with steamed green vegetables (try tenderstem broccoli, purple sprouting broccoli or sugar snap peas) (total GL = 10)
VARIATIONS use smoked trout instead of salmon, and add some petits pois instead of the courgette
ALLERGY SUITABILITY gluten, wheat free

MAINTENANCE PHASE
serve with 40g wholemeal pasta (dry weight) or 3 small boiled baby new potatoes (total GL = 15)

Pesto-crusted salmon

The strong, herby flavours of pesto work brilliantly with salmon –
and you can ring the changes with any of the other pesto recipes in
this book. An easy recipe if you are having friends round and don't
want the cooking to interrupt the conversation.

SERVES 2
1/2 tbsp olive oil
2 salmon fillets
2 portions of pesto (choose from the recipes on pages
    142–4 or use ready-made)

1 Preheat the oven to 180C/350F/Gas mark 4.
2 Grease a baking tray with the olive oil and place the salmon fillets
on it, spreading the pesto on top of them.
3 Bake for 18 minutes or until the flesh flakes easily when pressed.

Teriyaki salmon

Fiona's love affair with teriyaki sauce began at Yo! Sushi, where
they do an amazing teriyaki chicken. This version of the sauce is
lower in fat and sugar free but keeps all the flavours – and is a
doddle to cook.

SERVES 2
2 salmon fillets
2 portions of Teriyaki sauce (see page 157)

1 Preheat the oven to 190C/375F/Gas mark 5. Cut two large squares
of baking paper, each large enough to cover a fillet lying diagonally
across the middle of the paper when folded in half on the diagonal.
2 Marinate the salmon in the Teriyaki sauce for 30 minutes in the
fridge if you have time. (Don't worry if you don't – it will still work
but will simply lack the same depth of flavour.)
3 Place one salmon fillet and half of any remaining marinade liquid
in the centre of one piece of paper, then fold in half diagonally, corner
to corner, to make a triangle.
4 Starting from one end, gradually fold up the edges to seal them
an inch at a time, overlapping each fold slightly over the last to stop
it unravelling. By the time you reach the other end, the parcel should
be sealed (you can secure the last fold with a paperclip if you like,
or just tuck it underneath the parcel).
5 Repeat with the other fillet, place the two parcels on a baking tray
and bake for 25 minutes.
6 Unwrap the parcels carefully to avoid being burnt by the steam,
and place the fish on plates. Serve immediately.

Hot smoked salmon with crème fraîche and herb sauce

The tartness of crème fraîche contrasts well with the smoky taste of the fish. Ridiculously easy to make for a speedy supper.

SERVES 2
2 hot smoked salmon fillets
2 portions of Crème fraîche and herb sauce (see page 156)
Freshly ground black pepper

1 Gently heat the fish according to the pack instructions.
2 Meanwhile, make the sauce. Pour it over the fish and season with black pepper.

(GL) PER SERVING: 2

COOK'S NOTES
SERVING SUGGESTIONS (PER PERSON) serve with 3 small boiled baby new potatoes and steamed tenderstem, broccoli or mangetout (total (GL) = 11)
ALLERGY SUITABILITY gluten, wheat free

✓ **MAINTENANCE PHASE**
serve with 4 small boiled baby new potatoes or 1 small baked potato and Lemon and mint petits pois (see page 149) (total (GL) = 15)

Salmon and cherry tomato bake

Salmon fillets swimming in a creamy sauce with sweet, juicy cherry tomatoes – scrummy.

SERVES 2
1 tbsp olive oil
225g (8oz) cherry tomatoes
2 salmon fillets, boned
1½ tbsp low-fat crème fraîche
1 tbsp basil leaves, chopped or roughly torn
Freshly ground black pepper

1 Preheat the oven to 190C/375F/Gas mark 5.
2 Pour the olive oil into a shallow ovenproof dish (one that can also go on the hob). Place the whole cherry tomatoes around the salmon in the dish and cook for 25 minutes or until the fish is done, basting halfway through.
3 When the fish is cooked, place the dish on the hob and add the crème fraîche. Heat gently until it starts to bubble, then simmer for a few minutes until the sauce thickens.
4 Stir in the basil and season with black pepper.

(GL) PER SERVING: 4

COOK'S NOTES
SERVING SUGGESTION (PER PERSON) serve with half a small baked potato and a green salad (total (GL) = 11)
ALLERGY SUITABILITY gluten, wheat free

✓ **MAINTENANCE PHASE**
increase to a whole small baked potato and a large green salad (total (GL) = 15)

Hot smoked trout with pumpkin seed pesto and watercress open sandwich

Fiona devised this recipe for a competition, to showcase foods good for the skin. It's a firm favourite – delicious and full of essential fats and zinc.

SERVES 2
2 slices of thin pumpernickel style rye bread
1 tbsp pumpkin seed pesto (see page 143)
1 hot smoked trout fillet, flaked (checking for bones as you do so)
1 handful of watercress, roughly chopped
Freshly ground black pepper

1 Toast the rye bread (optional) and spread with the pesto.
2 Place the flaked fish on top and scatter with watercress.
3 Season with black pepper and serve.

PER SERVING: 6

COOK'S NOTES
SERVING SUGGESTION (PER PERSON) serve with a 4 GL starter or pudding (like Chocolate dipped nuts – see page 179) to total 10 GL
VARIATIONS use hot smoked salmon instead of trout, or normal smoked salmon or trout rather than hot smoked fish
ALLERGY SUITABILITY wheat, dairy free

MAINTENANCE PHASE
double up the quantities for 2 sandwiches per person, plus a 3 GL starter, drink or pudding to total 15 GL

Grilled trout with lemon and almonds

A dish with wonderfully complementary flavours, which is rich in valuable omega fatty acids.

SERVES 2
2 rainbow trout, gutted
Juice of 1 lemon
Low sodium salt or sea salt
Freshly ground black pepper
1 tbsp olive oil
2 tbsp flaked almonds

1 Season the inside of each fish with a good squeeze of lemon juice, a little salt and pepper. Rub the outside with the oil, then more lemon juice and pepper.
2 Grill under a moderate heat for 10 minutes, turning halfway through then sprinkle the almonds on top and return to the oven for a further 2 minutes (take care not to let the almonds burn).

PER SERVING: 1

COOK'S NOTES
SERVING SUGGESTION (PER PERSON) serve with simple flavours like green salad or steamed broccoli and 3 small boiled baby new potatoes (total GL = 10)
VARIATIONS omit the almonds if you don't like them or have a nut allergy
ALLERGY SUITABILITY gluten, wheat, dairy, yeast free

MAINTENANCE PHASE
increase to 4 small boiled baby new potatoes and serve with Baked fennel (see page 149) (total GL = 14)

Trout en papillote with lemon and garlic

Cooking en papillote, or in a parcel, is particularly successful with trout, as it protects the delicate essential fats while preserving the subtle flavours of the fish.

SERVES 2
2 medium-sized rainbow trout, gutted
2 cloves of garlic, crushed
Juice of 1 lemon
1 dsp fresh flat leaf parsley leaves, finely chopped
Low sodium salt or sea salt
Freshly ground black pepper

1 Preheat the oven to 180C/350F/Gas mark 4.

2 Cut 2 large squares of baking paper, each large enough to cover a fish lying diagonally across the middle of the paper when folded in half on the diagonal.

3 Season the inside of each fish with the garlic, lemon juice, parsley, salt and pepper.

4 Place each fish diagonally across one piece of baking paper, then fold in half on the diagonal, point to point, to make a triangle.

5 Starting at one end, gradually fold up the edges to seal them an inch at a time, overlapping each fold slightly over the last fold to stop it unravelling. By the time you reach the other end the parcel should be sealed (you can secure the last fold with a paperclip if you like, or just fold it underneath the parcel).

6 Repeat with the other fish. Place both parcels on a baking tray and bake for 25 minutes. Unwrap the parcels carefully to avoid being burnt by the steam, and place the fish on plates. Serve immediately.

PER SERVING: 1

COOK'S NOTES
SERVING SUGGESTION (PER PERSON) serve with 3 boiled baby new potatoes and rocket with a tomato and red onion salad (total = 9)
ALLERGY SUITABILITY gluten, wheat, dairy, yeast free

MAINTENANCE PHASE
serve with Roasted vegetables (see page 150) and 4 small boiled baby new potatoes (total = 16)

Smoked trout omelette

It's usually salmon you'll see partnered with eggs on breakfast menus, but smoked trout works just as well and makes a pleasant change. This is superfood for the brain, combining phospholipids from the egg and omega-3s from the fish – and plenty of protein to fill you up.

SERVES 1
2 medium eggs
Pinch of low sodium salt or sea salt
Freshly ground black pepper
1 slice smoked trout, chopped up
1 tbsp coconut oil or olive oil

1 Beat the eggs with the salt and pepper and smoked trout pieces.
2 Melt the oil in an omelette pan or medium-sized frying pan, then pour in the beaten egg mixture. Quickly stir the omelette around to allow the raw egg to come into contact with the pan base and start to set.
3 Let the omelette cook through until it is set at the edges and starting to set on top; this will take a couple of minutes. Then carefully insert a heat-proof spatula underneath and push it around the pan to detach the omelette. Tip the omelette out flat onto a plate, then slide it back into the pan to allow the other side to set – this will take only 30 seconds or so. Remove from the heat and serve.

GB **PER SERVING: 0**

COOK'S NOTES
SERVING SUGGESTION (PER PERSON) serve by itself and have 1½ thin slices toasted pumpernickel style rye bread or 1 medium slice wholemeal toast with peanut butter or pumpkin seed butter to follow, or serve the omelette on 1½ thin slices toasted pumpernickel style rye bread or 1 medium slice wholemeal toast with grilled tomatoes (total GB = 9)
VARIATIONS make with smoked salmon and chives, Parmesan and pumpkin seeds, roasted pepper and artichoke, peas and ham, courgettes and cherry tomatoes, or onions and mushrooms
ALLERGY SUITABILITY gluten, wheat, dairy free

✓ **MAINTENANCE PHASE**
serve with 2 medium slices wholemeal toast or 2 thin slices toasted pumpernickel style rye bread with 1 grilled tomato (total GB = 12)

Hot smoked trout with flageolet beans in white sauce

An impressive dinner party dish that tastes fantastic, yet takes minutes to prepare. It's served with tenderstem broccoli – young broccoli stems packed with nutrients like vitamin C and antioxidants.

SERVES 2
2 portions of Flageolet beans in white sauce (see page 154)
2 handfuls of tenderstem broccoli
2 hot smoked trout fillets (approximately 75g/3oz each)
Freshly ground black pepper
2 sprigs of fresh flat leaf parsley

1 Make the Flageolet beans in white sauce according to the recipe.
2 Meanwhile, steam the tenderstem for 3 to 5 minutes until tender to the bite. Don't overcook it as you don't want to lose all the nutrients.
3 Place the tenderstem and trout on each plate and top with the beans in sauce. Season with plenty of black pepper and a sprig of parsley.

GB **PER SERVING: 10**

COOK'S NOTES
VARIATIONS replace the trout with hot smoked salmon or cooked smoked haddock. Use normal broccoli or purple sprouting broccoli if you can't get tenderstem
ALLERGY SUITABILITY gluten, wheat, dairy free

✓ **MAINTENANCE PHASE**
serve with a 5 GB starter or pudding to total 15 GB

Red lentil and smoked mackerel kedgeree

This cross between kedgeree and lentil curry is so moreish that you will have to stop yourself eating it all from the pan before you serve it. The lentils are very low GL, while mackerel is an excellent source of omega-3s. You can double this recipe and store in the fridge for up to 2 days.

SERVES 2

½ tsp turmeric
1 tsp medium curry powder
1 tbsp coconut oil or olive oil
2 cloves of garlic, crushed
1 onion, chopped
250g (9oz) red lentils, well rinsed and drained
690ml (1 pt 3fl. oz) cold water
4 tsp Marigold Reduced Salt Vegetable Bouillon powder
1 hardboiled egg (8 minutes), cooled, then peeled and sliced
2 small smoked mackerel fillets (75g/3oz in total), skinned
    and flaked into pieces (checking for bones as you do so)

1 Dry-fry the turmeric and curry powder for 1 minute in a large frying pan.
2 Add the oil and garlic and fry for 30 seconds, then add the onion and sweat until it softens.
3 Place the lentils, water and bouillon powder in the pan and boil, uncovered, for 10 minutes.
4 Cover and simmer for 15 to 20 minutes until the lentils are soft to the bite. Stir in the egg slices and flaked fish at the end before serving.

GL PER SERVING: 4

COOK'S NOTES
SERVING SUGGESTION (PER PERSON) serve hot or cold. Add a side salad or steamed green beans or cauliflower for extra vegetables (total GL = 6) and have a 4 GL starter or pudding to total 10 GL, or serve with 45g brown basmati rice (dry weight) (total GL = 11)
VARIATIONS delicious without the egg and fish, as a plain dahl or lentil curry
ALLERGY SUITABILITY gluten, wheat, dairy free

✓ MAINTENANCE PHASE
serve with 60g brown basmati rice (dry weight) and a green salad (total GL = 15)

Smoked mackerel, leek and bean soup

A warming and filling soup and a balanced meal on its own, with fibre from the leeks and plenty of protein from the beans and fish. You can double this recipe and store in the fridge for up to 2 days.

SERVES 2
1 tsp coconut oil or olive oil
2 cloves of garlic, crushed
2 large leeks (300g/11oz trimmed weight), trimmed
  and well rinsed then sliced
600ml (1pt) boiling water
3 tsp Marigold Reduced Salt Vegetable Bouillon powder
1 x 410g can cannellini beans, rinsed and drained
1 smoked mackerel fillet (approximately 75g/3oz),
  skin removed
Freshly ground black pepper

1 Heat the oil in a pan and sauté the garlic for 30 seconds.
2 Add the leeks, cover and sweat for 3 minutes until they start to soften.
3 Pour the water and bouillon powder into the pan and stir, then cover and simmer for a couple of minutes.
4 Add the beans and blend with a handheld blender until fairly smooth.
5 Flake the fish, checking for bones, and stir into the soup before seasoning with black pepper.

Smoked mackerel salad

Peppered and smoked mackerel fillets add a smoky, salty flavour to enliven the cannellini beans, while providing plenty of omega-3s.

SERVES 2
2 peppered smoked mackerel fillets (approximately
  75g/3oz each), skinned, flaked and checked for bones
1 x 410g can cannellini beans, rinsed and drained
10 cm (4 in) chunk of cucumber, quartered lengthways
  then sliced horizontally into chunks
1 red onion, diced
5–6 cherry tomatoes, quartered
6 Kalamata olives, pitted and halved

DRESSING
1 tbsp olive oil
2 tsp lemon juice
Freshly ground black pepper

1 Mix together all of the salad ingredients.
2 Make the dressing and toss through the salad.

Salade niçoise

A flavour-packed low-GL alternative to the classic French dish. As tuna can be high in mercury and shouldn't be eaten more than once a month, here, we've given you the option of using eggs and anchovies (you can still use tuna, of course – see Cook's Notes for amounts). Mixed pulses take the place of the traditional boiled potatoes to lower the GL and make a tasty and interesting change.

SERVES 2

1 Romaine lettuce, washed well, dried and torn into bite-sized pieces
6 spring onions, sliced on the diagonal
6 black olives, pitted and halved
2 eggs, hardboiled (8 minutes), shelled and chopped into smallish chunks
4 anchovies in oil, drained on kitchen towel and sliced into 1cm strips
2 large ripe tomatoes, chopped
Freshly ground black pepper
1 x 410g can mixed pulses, rinsed and drained
225g (8oz) cooked French green beans, rinsed and drained well to remove any salty water

FOR THE DRESSING

2 tbsp extra virgin olive oil
2 tsp lemon juice
1/2 clove garlic, crushed
Freshly ground black pepper
Pinch of xylitol or caster sugar

1 Toss all of the salad ingredients together.
2 Pour over the dressing and toss again, gently.

GL PER SERVING: 7

COOK'S NOTES

SERVING SUGGESTION (PER PERSON) have a 3 GL starter, pudding or drink (like St Clement's smoothie – see page 182) to total 10 GL

VARIATIONS replace the mixed pulses with pinto or borlotti beans or 3 boiled baby new potatoes per person. Replace the anchovies and egg with a 185g can tuna steak in spring water or olive oil, drained. Vegetarians could leave out the anchovies and add another egg per person for extra protein, plus a few more olives to replace the fish

ALLERGY SUITABILITY gluten, wheat free

MAINTENANCE PHASE

serve with 3 small boiled baby new potatoes (in addition to the mixed pulses in the recipe) (total GL = 14)

Mediterranean pasta

If you hanker after macaroni cheese or spaghetti carbonara, you'll love this recipe. You can make this with tuna, as an occasional treat, or substitute chicken goujons if you like. You can double this recipe and store in the fridge for up to 2 days.

SERVES 2
125g (5oz) wholemeal pasta
1 x 185g can tuna in spring water, drained
10 sun-blush tomato quarters (jarred or from the deli),
   drained and chopped
1 tbsp black olives, pitted and halved
300ml (½ pt) skimmed milk, soya milk or nut milk
2 tsp Marigold Reduced Salt Vegetable Bouillon powder
1 tsp dried Italian herbs
1 tbsp cornflour mixed with 2 tbsp water until smooth
Freshly ground black pepper
1 tbsp fresh basil, finely chopped

1 Cook the pasta according to the pack instructions and drain, then stir in the tuna, sun blush tomatoes and olives.
2 Next, make the white sauce by pouring the milk into a pan and stirring in the bouillon powder and dried herbs. Add the cornflour liquid and whisk for 3 to 5 minutes over a gentle heat until the sauce is thick and smooth.
3 Pour the sauce over the pasta, season with black pepper and sprinkle the basil over the top, mixing gently before serving.

Tuna steak with sesame quinoa

Grilled tuna steak is wonderful with this full-flavoured, Oriental-style quinoa. Remember that the mercury contamination of tuna means you should make it an occasional treat.

SERVES 2

140g (just over 5oz) quinoa
360ml (12floz) boiling water
1 tsp Marigold Reduced Salt Vegetable Bouillon powder
2 fresh tuna steaks
3–4 tbsp fresh or frozen petits pois
2 tsp sesame oil
1 tbsp tamari (wheat-free soy sauce) or soy sauce
2 tsp lemon juice
1 large carrot, julienned
6 spring onions, finely sliced
Freshly ground black pepper

1 Cook the quinoa by placing it in a pan with the water and bouillon powder. Bring back to the boil. Cover and simmer for around 13 minutes, or until all the water has been absorbed and the quinoa is soft and fluffy.
2 Meanwhile, grill the tuna steaks under a moderate heat for 10 to 12 minutes, turning halfway through.
3 Add the peas to the cooked quinoa, stir through, then remove from the heat (they will cook or soften slightly in the residual warmth).
4 Combine the quinoa with all the other ingredients, tossing thoroughly to mix all the flavours and allow the quinoa to soak up the liquid.
5 Serve each steak on a bed of quinoa.

PER SERVING: 5

COOK'S NOTES
SERVING SUGGESTION (PER PERSON) serve with a 5 GL starter or pudding to total 10 GL
VARIATIONS serve the sesame quinoa with other fish such as salmon, haddock or mackerel
ALLERGY SUITABILITY gluten, wheat, dairy free (use tamari instead of soy if you cannot eat wheat)

MAINTENANCE PHASE
serve with both a 5 GL starter and a pudding to total 15 GL – or cut out the starter and have a more decadent pudding (such as Chocolate hazelnut mousse – see page 162) to total 16 GL

PER SERVING: 8

SERVING SUGGESTION (PER PERSON)
serve with a mixed salad of green
leaves, tomatoes and red onion
(total GL = 9)
VARIATION replace the fish with
cooked chicken, chopped ham,
white fish or prawns. Use peas and
asparagus instead of the tomatoes
and olives for an early summer
version
ALLERGY SUITABILITY gluten, wheat,
dairy free

MAINTENANCE PHASE
serve with the salad as above plus a
6 GL starter or pudding to total 15 GL

Mediterranean tomato risotto with tuna

This risotto uses brown basmati rice instead of high-GL Arborio rice.
The fresh cherry tomatoes and sun-dried tomato paste provide a rich
sauce for the rice. Because it's advisable to limit your tuna intake,
you can vary this recipe by using other sources of protein, such as
marinated anchovies or cooked chicken.

SERVES 2
150g (just over 5oz) brown basmati rice
2 tsp Marigold Reduced Salt Vegetable Bouillon powder
    dissolved in 210ml (7 fl. oz) water
2 tbsp sun-dried tomato paste
2 handfuls of cherry tomatoes, halved or 2 tbsp canned
    chopped tomatoes
2 tbsp dry black olives, pitted and chopped
4 spring onions, finely sliced on the diagonal
1 x 185g can tuna in spring water, drained, or 50g (2oz) marinated
    drained anchovies (from the deli or look out for marinated
    anchovies in the chiller cabinet)
1 tbsp fresh basil leaves or chives, roughly torn or chopped
Freshly ground black pepper

1 Bring the rice to the boil with the bouillon liquid, then cover and
simmer for around 15 to 20 minutes until the water is absorbed and
the rice is al dente.
2 Stir in the sun-dried tomato paste, cherry tomatoes or canned
tomatoes, olives and onions and continue to cook, stirring, until the
cherry tomatoes start to soften and break down.
3 Stir in the fish, sprinkle with herbs and season with black pepper.
Serve immediately.

Anchovy and tomato pasta sauce

A rich Mediterranean sauce for pasta. Anchovies are rich in omega-3 fatty acids but relatively low in heavy metal contamination. The fresh, marinated type from delis are infinitely preferable to the canned or jarred ones.

SERVES 2

3 good tbsp good quality tomato-based pasta sauce plus 1 tbsp water
2 handfuls of cherry tomatoes, halved
2 tbsp black olives, pitted and roughly chopped
50g (2oz) fresh anchovy fillets (from the deli or look out for marinated anchovies in the chiller cabinet)
Freshly ground black pepper

1 Put the tomato sauce, tomatoes and olives in a pan and simmer until the tomatoes start to soften.
2 Stir in the anchovies, season generously with black pepper and serve over wholemeal pasta.

GL PER SERVING: 4

COOK'S NOTES

SERVING SUGGESTION (PER PERSON) serve with 40g wholemeal pasta (dry weight) and a large salad (total GL = 11)

VARIATION replace the anchovies with canned tuna in spring water or olive oil (drain, then stir in). Add some fresh herbs such as basil, roughly torn and sprinkled over the top after cooking

ALLERGY SUITABILITY gluten, wheat, dairy free

MAINTENANCE PHASE increase the wholemeal pasta serving size to 55g (dry weight) and again serve with a large salad (total GL = 15)

VEGETARIAN

One of the joys of the Holford Diet is its emphasis on vegetarian food – which is not only the backbone of many world cuisines but a wonderfully healthy dietary option. Along with the staggering array of vegetables we're now seeing in supermarkets, the variety of pulses, seeds and nuts and grains to be found makes for a deliciously varied nutritional and taste palette. So you'll find that there's a lot to play with in this section, from inventive ways with cheeses like halloumi, to jazzed-up classics such as stuffed peppers, lentil curries and tabboulleh. Bear in mind, too, that most of the meat and fish recipes in the preceding sections can be adjusted to your needs – smoked tofu is an excellent alternative.

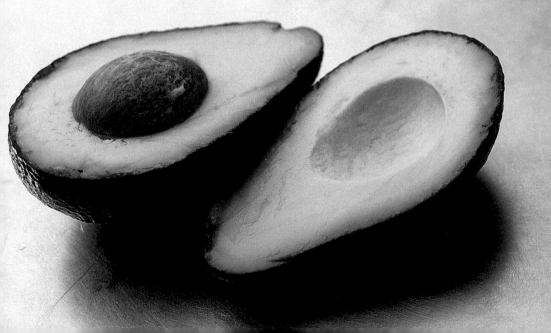

Greek salad

Ideal for lunch or a picnic on a hot day, this classic salad is full of summer flavours and rich in antioxidants from the red onion and ripe tomatoes. You can double this recipe and store in the fridge for up to 3 days.

SERVES 2
1 medium red onion, halved then thinly sliced
3 medium tomatoes, chopped into chunks
15cm (6in) chunk of cucumber, quartered lengthways then chopped into chunks
1½ tbsp Kalamata olives, pitted and halved
150g (just over 5oz) feta cheese
Freshly ground black pepper

FOR THE DRESSING
1½ tbsp extra virgin olive oil (if you can, use oil pressed from Greek Kalamata olives to complement the olives in the salad)
1 tbsp white wine vinegar
3/4 tsp dried oregano
Freshly ground black pepper

1 Put the vegetables and olives in a salad bowl, pour over the dressing and toss gently.
2 Crumble the feta on top and lightly toss through the vegetables.
3 Season with black pepper and chill lightly or serve immediately.

GL PER SERVING: 3

COOK'S NOTES
SERVING SUGGESTION (PER PERSON)
serve on a generous bed of crispy lettuce like little gem, Romaine or Cos with 3 small boiled baby potatoes or 70g quinoa (dry weight) (total GL =10)
ALLERGY SUITABILITY gluten, wheat free

MAINTENANCE PHASE
serve with lettuce, as above, and 1 wholemeal pitta bread (total GL =13)

Feta and flageolet bean salad

Another superquick dish for a summer's day. Delicate green flageolet beans and rich, tangy feta are perfect partners – and the beans also contain phytoestrogens that help balance hormones. You can double this recipe and store in the fridge for up to 3 days.

SERVES 2
1 x 410g can flageolet beans, rinsed and drained
100g (4oz) feta cheese, cut into small cubes or crumbled
4 spring onions, finely sliced on the diagonal
Juice of ½ a lemon
1 tbsp olive oil
1 tbsp fresh flat leaf parsley leaves, finely chopped
Freshly ground black pepper

Mix together all of the ingredients and chill lightly or serve immediately.

GL PER SERVING: 7

COOK'S NOTES
SERVING SUGGESTION (PER PERSON)
serve on a generous bed of crispy Little Gem or Romaine lettuce with a 3 GL starter, pudding or drink to total 10 GL, or serve with 35g quinoa (dry weight) for a 10 GL meal
VARIATIONS adjust the seasoning (lemon juice, spring onions and herbs) according to taste
ALLERGY SUITABILITY gluten, wheat free

MAINTENANCE PHASE
increase the quinoa serving to 70g (dry weight) and serve with a large green salad (total GL = 15)

Sun-blush tomato and black olive chickpea salad

This strong-flavoured salad combines Middle Eastern and Mediterranean flavours very successfully. You can double this recipe and store in the fridge for up to 3 days.

SERVES 2

1 x 410g can chickpeas, rinsed and drained
1 dsp sun blush tomatoes in oil, chopped
   (reserve the oil as a dressing)
1 dsp 'dry' black olives (packed without oil or brine),
   pitted and chopped
4 spring onions, finely sliced on the diagonal
1 tsp fresh flat leaf parsley, finely chopped
1 dsp lemon juice
1 dsp tahini
Freshly ground black pepper
1 dsp oil reserved from the sun blush tomatoes
   (or plain extra virgin olive oil)

Mix together all of the ingredients and chill lightly or serve immediately.

GL PER SERVING: 8

COOK'S NOTES
SERVING SUGGESTION (PER PERSON)
serve with a green salad and a slice of Sesame cornbread (see page 129) or a cooked chicken breast, fish fillet or cubed smoked tofu to make a main meal (total GL = 10)
ALLERGY SUITABILITY gluten, wheat, dairy free

✓ **MAINTENANCE PHASE**
serve with 70g (dry weight) quinoa and a green salad (total GL = 15)

COOK'S NOTES
SERVING SUGGESTION (PER PERSON)
serve warm with a rocket and
lamb's leaf salad (total **GL** = 10)
VARIATIONS the roasted chickpeas
make an excellent snack on their
own. Store in an airtight container
in the fridge.
ALLERGY SUITABILITY gluten, wheat,
dairy, yeast free

✔ **MAINTENANCE PHASE**
serve with a 5 **GL** starter or pudding
to total 15 **GL**

Roasted chickpea and lemon taboulleh

When roasted, chickpeas develop a lovely chewy yet crunchy texture. Enlivened with lemon and spices, they are delicious in this taboulleh salad. You can double this recipe and store in the fridge for up to 3 days.

SERVES 2
140g (just over 5oz) quinoa, rinsed and drained
390ml (13fl. oz) water
1 tsp Marigold Reduced Salt Vegetable Bouillon powder
1 x 410g can chickpeas, rinsed and drained
2 tbsp olive oil
1 tsp ground cumin
1 clove of garlic, crushed
Finely grated zest of $^1/_2$ a lemon and juice of the whole lemon
1 tbsp sesame seeds
2 tbsp fresh flat leaf parsley leaves, chopped
Freshly ground black pepper

1 Preheat the oven to 200C/400F/Gas mark 6.
2 Cook the quinoa by putting it in a pan with the water and bouillon powder and bringing all to a boil. Cover and simmer for 13 minutes or until the water is absorbed and the quinoa grains are soft and fluffy.
3 Meanwhile, toss the chickpeas in a tablespoon of the oil and the cumin, garlic, lemon zest and juice and sesame seeds.
4 Tip the chickpeas into a roasting tin and cook for 30 minutes, shaking halfway through (the sesame seeds should turn golden but not burn).
5 Mix the chickpeas into the cooked quinoa with the parsley, black pepper and the remaining tablespoon of oil.

Stuffed peppers

These delicious stuffed peppers first appeared in *The Holford Low-GL Diet*, but they're so good we couldn't leave them out here. A rich stuffing with pine nuts, basil and mushrooms partners the sweet peppers brilliantly.

SERVES 2

1 tsp olive oil (for greasing)
2 large red peppers
1 tbsp coconut oil or olive oil
1 medium onion, finely chopped
2 cloves of garlic, crushed
150g (just over 5oz) mushrooms, cleaned with a brush or wiped with kitchen towel and sliced
1 tsp Marigold Reduced Salt Vegetable Bouillon powder
2–3 tbsp water
100g (4oz) brown basmati rice, cooked
1 tbsp pine nuts
Handful of fresh basil, chopped
Low-sodium salt or sea salt
Freshly ground black pepper

1 Preheat the oven to 200C/400F/Gas mark 6 and lightly grease a baking tray with the teaspoon of oil.
2 Cut the top off the peppers (reserving the lid), remove the seeds and pith and slice off the bulbous bit inside the pepper that sits below the stalk and contains most of the seeds.
3 Heat the remaining oil in a sauté pan and gently fry the onion and garlic for 2 minutes. Add the chopped mushrooms and bouillon powder and fry for a further 2 to 3 minutes.
4 In a large bowl, combine this mixture with the cooked rice, pine nuts and basil and season with a little salt and black pepper.
5 Stuff the peppers with the mixture and place the tops back on.
6 Place on the baking tray and bake for 35 minutes. Serve immediately.

GL PER SERVING: 9

COOK'S NOTES
SERVING SUGGESTION (PER PERSON) this is a complete meal on its own, but looks very nice served with a salad of mixed leaves, tomatoes and red onion (total GL = 10)
ALLERGY SUITABILITY gluten, wheat, dairy, yeast free

MAINTENANCE PHASE
serve with the salad as above plus a 5 GL starter or pudding to total 15 GL

COOK'S NOTES
SERVING SUGGESTION (PER PERSON)
serve as a 5 GL snack or starter with
some green leaves like Little Gem or
Cos, or with 3 small boiled baby new
potatoes for an 11 GL main meal
ALLERGY SUITABILITY gluten,
wheat free

✓ **MAINTENANCE PHASE**
serve with 1 toasted wholemeal pitta
bread and lettuce (total GL = 15)

Greek stuffed peppers

A new take on stuffed peppers, here the filling is added after
cooking. The crunchy, fresh Greek salad is a wonderful contrast
to the soft, sweet peppers. These can be served warm or chilled.

SERVES 2
1 tsp olive oil (for greasing)
2 red peppers
100g (4oz) feta cheese, crumbled
1/2 a medium red onion, diced
1 tbsp Kalamata olives, pitted and halved
2 medium ripe tomatoes, chopped into chunks
10cm (4in) chunk of cucumber, halved lengthways then chopped
   horizontally into chunks
Freshly ground black pepper

FOR THE DRESSING
1 tbsp extra virgin olive oil
1/2 tbsp white wine vinegar
1/2 tsp dried oregano
Freshly ground black pepper

1 Preheat the oven to 200C/400F/Gas mark 6. Lightly grease
a baking tray with the teaspoon of oil.
2 Cut the tops off the peppers (reserving the lids), remove the seeds
and pith and slice off the bulbous bit inside the pepper that sits below
the stalk and contains most of the seeds.
3 Place the peppers upright on the baking tray and put the tops
back on. Roast for 25 minutes, then drain off the water that will
have accumulated in the peppers.
4 Toss all of the salad ingredients together, pour over the dressing,
then toss again gently. Spoon into the roasted peppers and serve
warm or lightly chilled.

Avocado gazpacho

Chilled soups are fast and nutrient-rich and ideal for entertaining, as they are easy to prepare in advance. Serve this deliciously fresh-tasting gazpacho straight from the fridge on a hot day.

SERVES 2

1/2 a small red onion, diced
1/2 a red pepper, diced
1 stick celery, sliced
5cm (2in) chunk of cucumber, quartered lengthways then finely sliced horizontally into small triangles
Good handful of cherry tomatoes
1/2 clove of garlic, crushed
2 tsp mild red chilli, deseeded and finely chopped
300ml (1/2 pt) tomato juice or V8 (vegetable juice)
Juice of 1 lime
1 dsp of fresh coriander, finely chopped
1 ripe avocado, peeled and chopped
Freshly ground black pepper

1 Stir all the ingredients except for the avocado and pepper together.
2 Using a handheld blender or food processor, pulse the mixture to roughly blend it, but leave it fairly chunky for texture.
3 Stir in the avocado, sprinkle with the pepper and chill till ready to serve.

GL PER SERVING: 8

COOK'S NOTES
SERVING SUGGESTION (PER PERSON) serve with the Hummus soufflé (see page 83) as a starter to total 10 GL
VARIATIONS vary the vegetables used – add more chilli and onions if you like it hotter, or use roasted peppers instead of raw ones
ALLERGY SUITABILITY gluten, wheat, dairy, yeast free

✓ MAINTENANCE PHASE
serve with the Hummus soufflé (see page 83) as a starter and have a 5 GL pudding to total 15 GL

Leek and potato soup

A thick, satisfying soup, which has a relatively low GL because we've substituted blended cannellini beans for some of the potatoes. And it's a complete, balanced meal. You can triple this recipe and freeze the remainder, or store in the fridge for up to 4 days.

SERVES 2

1 tsp coconut oil or olive oil
2 cloves garlic, crushed
2 large leeks (300g/11oz trimmed weight), trimmed and well rinsed, then sliced
2 medium or 3 small baby new potatoes (approximately 75g/3oz), unpeeled and cubed
600ml (1pt) boiling water
3 tsp Marigold Reduced Salt Vegetable Bouillon powder
1 x 410g can cannellini beans, rinsed and drained
Freshly ground black pepper

1 Heat the oil in a pan and sauté the garlic for 30 seconds.
2 Add the leeks, cover and sweat for 3 minutes until they start to soften.
3 Tip the potatoes, water and bouillon powder into the pan and stir, then cover and simmer for 15 minutes.
4 Add the beans and blend with a handheld blender until fairly smooth. Season with black pepper.

GL PER SERVING: 11

COOK'S NOTES
ALLERGY SUITABILITY gluten, wheat, dairy, yeast free

✓ MAINTENANCE PHASE
serve with 2 rough oat cakes (total GL = 15) or with a 4 GL starter or pudding to total 15 GL

Chestnut and butterbean soup

An all-time favourite at Fiona's cookery demonstrations. Chestnuts have the lowest fat content of all nuts and a pleasantly sweet flavour that goes well with the smooth texture of the blended butterbeans. This is fast, easy and deliciously filling. You can triple this recipe and freeze the remainder, or store in the fridge for up to 4 days.

SERVES 2

200g (7oz) cooked and peeled chestnuts (available vacuum-packed in boxes, cans or jars)
1 x 410g can of butterbeans, rinsed and drained
1 medium white onion, chopped
1 large carrot, peeled and chopped
3 tsp Marigold Reduced Salt Vegetable Bouillon powder dissolved in 600ml (1 pint) water
Freshly ground black pepper

1 Place all the ingredients (except for a handful of the chestnuts and the pepper) in a saucepan, place a lid on it and bring to the boil. Simmer gently for 15 to 20 minutes.
2 Purée the soup in a blender or food processor until smooth and season with the black pepper.
3 Sprinkle the reserved chestnuts on top.

GL PER SERVING: 12

COOK'S NOTES
ALLERGY SUITABILITY
gluten, wheat, dairy, yeast free

✓ MAINTENANCE PHASE
serve with 1 rough oat cake (total GL = 15)

Sesame cornbread

This is a simply brilliant recipe. It takes just 30 minutes to make and bake, and it's perfect for when you crave bread. Enjoy it warm and crumbly straight from the oven.

SERVES 3

75g (3oz) polenta flour or cornmeal
75g (3oz) sesame seeds, finely ground
1 tbsp poppy seeds
½ tsp salt
3 tsp baking powder
1 dsp coconut oil
1 large egg, beaten
150 ml (¼ pt) skimmed milk, soya milk or nut milk
1 tbsp sesame seeds, for sprinkling on top

1 Preheat the oven to 200C/400F/Gas mark 6. Line a small baking tray (if you only have a standard baking tray measuring 23cm x 32cm (9in x 12in) don't worry; although the mixture will only fill half the tin it holds its shape well).
2 Mix the polenta or cornmeal with the ground sesame seeds, poppy seeds, salt and baking powder in a bowl.
3 Heat the coconut oil gently in a pan. Pour into a bowl and mix with the beaten egg and milk.
4 Stir the wet and dry ingredients together and pour into the prepared baking tray, smoothing out into a level, even shape.
5 Sprinkle the sesame seeds on top and bake in the oven for 15 minutes, until the centre is firm and springy to the touch. Lift the bread out of the tray by holding the paper and tap its base - the bread will sound hollow if cooked.
6 Slice into 6 and serve warm from the oven, or allow to cool on a wire rack and store unsliced in an airtight container (Sesame cornbread is better eaten the day of or the day after cooking).

PER SERVING: 1 (2 SLICES)

COOK'S NOTES
SERVING SUGGESTION (PER PERSON) serve with a bowl of Vegetable chilli (see page 131), or with a bowl of soup or salad
VARIATIONS experiment with different herbs and spices such as chilli, Italian mixed herbs or chives
ALLERGY SUITABILITY gluten, wheat, dairy, yeast free

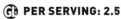

Pumpernickel croutons

For anyone who likes to have something to fish for in their soup, pumpernickel style rye bread has a chewy, nutty texture and flavour, making it excellent for croutons. This way you avoid the wheat and fat of the usual kind, and turn your bowl of soup into a complete meal.

SERVES 2

1 thin slice pumpernickel style rye bread

Toast the bread, cut it into bite-sized squares and scatter them between two bowls of soup. Serve.

PER SERVING: 2.5

COOK'S NOTES
ALLERGY SUITABILITY gluten, wheat, dairy free

COOK'S NOTES
SERVING SUGGESTION (PER PERSON)
serve with 35g quinoa (dry weight)
(total GL = 10.5)
VARIATIONS omit the almonds if
preferred, or if you have a nut
allergy
ALLERGY SUITABILITY gluten,
wheat, dairy, yeast free

MAINTENANCE PHASE
serve with 45g brown basmati rice
(dry weight) (total GL = 14)

Chickpea curry

You can throw together this tasty curry in about 5 minutes flat, using nothing but storecupboard staples. And it's bursting with valuable nutrients, from the antioxidants in the garlic, onion and curry powder to the calcium and magnesium in the almonds and the phytoestrogens in the chickpeas. You can double this recipe and freeze the remainder, or store in the fridge for up to 3 days.

SERVES 2
1 tsp coconut oil or olive oil
2 cloves of garlic, crushed
1 onion, diced
2 tsp curry powder
300ml (1/2 pt) water
2 tsp Marigold Reduced Salt Vegetable Bouillon powder
2 tbsp tomato purée
1 x 410g can chickpeas, rinsed and drained
2 tbsp ground almonds

1 Heat the oil in a large frying pan or wok and fry the garlic and onion for 2 minutes.
2 Add the curry powder and cook until the onion softens.
3 Pour in the water and add the bouillon powder, tomato purée, chickpeas and ground almonds. Simmer and stir for a minute or so to let the mixture thicken.

Vegetable chilli

Packed with beans, vegetables and spices, this hearty vegetarian chilli has enough heat and texture to ensure you don't notice the absence of meat. It serves 4, so you can have it again the next night (the flavour improves if left to develop in the fridge – you can keep it there for up to 3 days) or freeze the leftovers.

SERVES 4

2 tsp coconut oil or olive oil
1 onion, diced
2 cloves of garlic, crushed
1 pepper, diced
1 tsp ground cumin
1 tsp crushed chilli flakes
1 tsp chilli powder
250g (9oz) mushrooms, cleaned with a brush or wiped
  with kitchen towel and sliced
1 x 400g can chopped tomatoes
3 tbsp tomato purée
1 x 410g can kidney beans, rinsed and drained
1 x 410g can borlotti beans, rinsed and drained
3 tsp Marigold Reduced Salt Vegetable Bouillon powder

1 Heat the oil in a pan and fry the onion and garlic for 2 minutes.
2 Add the pepper and spices and cover to sweat for 5 minutes, until the peppers soften.
3 Add the mushrooms and cook for a minute until they soften.
4 Tip in the chopped tomatoes, tomato purée, beans and bouillon powder, stir, then cover and simmer for 5 minutes.

PER SERVING: 6

COOK'S NOTES
SERVING SUGGESTION (PER PERSON) delicious with 35g quinoa (dry weight) (total GL = 9.5)
VARIATIONS vary the beans used – pinto beans or black-eye beans would also work well
ALLERGY SUITABILITY gluten, wheat, dairy, yeast free

MAINTENANCE PHASE
serve with 60g brown basmati rice (dry weight) (total GL = 16)

COOK'S NOTES
SERVING SUGGESTION (PER PERSON)
serve with 35g quinoa (dry weight)
(total **G** = 10.5)
VARIATIONS you can substitute any
kind of bean or lentil for the borlotti
beans. Pinto or kidney beans would
work well
ALLERGY SUITABILITY gluten, wheat,
dairy, yeast free

✓ **MAINTENANCE PHASE**
serve with 70g quinoa (dry weight)
(total **G** = 14)

Bean-stuffed aubergines

A rich, tomatoey stuffing brings the baked aubergine to life. Bursting with antioxidants from the onions, garlic, mushrooms and tomatoes, this would make a good, simple supper for friends – just double or triple the recipe.

SERVES 2
1 medium aubergine
2 tsp coconut oil or olive oil
2 cloves of garlic, crushed
2 red onions, diced
100g (4oz) button mushrooms, cleaned with a brush or wiped with
    kitchen towel and sliced
1 red pepper, deseeded and chopped fairly small
200g (7oz) tomato passata
1/2 x 410g can borlotti beans, rinsed and drained
1 tsp herbes de Provence
1 tsp Marigold Reduced Salt Vegetable Bouillon powder
Low-sodium salt or sea salt
Freshly ground black pepper
1 tsp olive oil (for brushing the aubergine)

1 Preheat the oven to 190C/375F/Gas mark 5.
2 Cut the aubergine in half and scoop out the flesh with a teaspoon to use in the stuffing, taking care not to puncture the skin. Put the shells to one side.
3 For the stuffing, heat the oil in a pan and cook the garlic for 30 seconds or so before adding the onions and letting them sweat and soften for a couple of minutes.
4 Add the mushrooms, reserved aubergine flesh and chopped pepper and cook for a few minutes or so until they soften slightly (this takes around 10 minutes in total).
5 Finally add the tomato passata, beans, herbs, bouillon powder and seasoning, stir and let the mixture simmer for 2 minutes or so.
6 Brush the outside of the reserved aubergine shells with the teaspoon of olive oil and place in a roasting tin, then stuff the shells with the filling. (If you have any left over, it's delicious with baked potatoes or pasta.) Cover the roasting tin with kitchen foil and bake for 40 to 45 minutes, until the aubergine is tender.

Peter's Mediterranean bean feast

This recipe was invented by the father of Fiona's boyfriend Nicholas, who serves it to any vegetarians he has to feed. Despite Peter being a devout meat eater himself, his recipe is seriously delicious.

SERVES 2

1 tsp olive oil
1 red onion, diced
1 x 410g can mixed pulses, drained and rinsed
2 tbsp good quality tomato-based pasta sauce
4 marinated artichoke hearts from a jar or the deli (optional)
Handful of black olives, pitted and roughly chopped
Freshly ground black pepper, to taste
Handful of fresh basil leaves, torn

1 Heat the oil in a saucepan and gently fry the onion for 1 to 2 minutes, just to take the raw edge off.
2 Add the mixed pulses, tomato sauce, artichoke hearts (if using) and olives, and stir.
3 Season with black pepper, remove from the heat and add the basil leaves. Allow to sit for a while if possible to let the flavours develop.

PER SERVING: 7

COOK'S NOTES
SERVING SUGGESTION (PER PERSON) delicious served warm or cold with 35g quinoa (dry weight) and a large green salad (total GL = 10.5)
VARIATIONS omit the artichoke hearts if you like
ALLERGY SUITABILITY gluten, wheat, dairy free

MAINTENANCE PHASE serve with 70g quinoa (dry weight) and salad (total GL = 15)

Borlotti Bolognese

This is a mouthwatering vegan alternative to spag bol, crammed with fibre and the antioxidant lycopene from the cooked tomatoes. It can be prepared in batches and frozen for convenience.

SERVES 2

2 tsp coconut oil or olive oil
2 cloves of garlic, crushed
1 onion, chopped
100g (4oz) button mushrooms, cleaned with a brush or wiped with kitchen towel and sliced
1½ tsp Marigold Reduced Salt Vegetable Bouillon powder
1 tsp herbes de Provence
1½ tbsp tomato purée
1 x 200g (7oz) can chopped tomatoes
1 x 410g can of borlotti beans, drained and rinsed
Low sodium salt or sea salt
Freshly ground black pepper

1 Heat the oil and cook the garlic and onion gently for 2 minutes, then add the mushrooms and cook till fairly soft (around 5 minutes).
2 Add the bouillon powder, dried herbs, tomato purée, canned tomatoes and beans, season and simmer for around 10 minutes to allow the vegetables to soften and the sauce to thicken.

PER SERVING: 7

COOK'S NOTES
SERVING SUGGESTION (PER PERSON) serve with 35g quinoa (dry weight) (total GL = 10.5)
VARIATIONS use kidney beans or pinto beans instead of borlotti beans
ALLERGY SUITABILITY gluten, wheat, dairy, yeast free

MAINTENANCE PHASE serve with 70g quinoa (dry weight) or 45g brown basmati rice (dry weight) (total GL = 15)

Asparagus and flageolet bean risotto

A gorgeous spring risotto, studded with green from the asparagus tips, flageolet beans and herbs. The brown basmati rice – which has the lowest GL score of all rice varieties – is just as creamy as Arborio, thanks to the addition of tahini white sauce.

SERVES 2

100g (4oz) brown basmati rice
2 tsp Marigold Reduced Salt Vegetable Bouillon powder dissolved
    in 210ml (7 fl. oz) water
100g (4oz) asparagus tips
1 x 410g can flageolet beans, rinsed and drained
2 handfuls of rocket, torn
1 dsp lemon juice
1 tbsp fresh flat leaf parsley leaves or chives, chopped
2 portions Tahini white sauce (see page 156)
Freshly ground black pepper, to taste

1 Bring the rice to the boil with the bouillon liquid, cover and simmer for around 15 to 20 minutes or until the water is absorbed and the rice is al dente.
2 While the rice is cooking, steam the asparagus for 7 to 8 minutes, until tender but not collapsing.
3 Mix in the flageolet beans, asparagus, rocket, lemon juice and herbs, stirring to allow the rocket to wilt slightly in the heat.
4 Make the Tahini white sauce according to the recipe instructions and stir into the risotto, ensuring that it is still piping hot. Season with black pepper, then serve.

Cashew and sesame quinoa

The sesame, tamari and cashews enliven this dish, while the raw veg provide extra crunch and vitamins and antioxidants. You can double this recipe and store in the fridge for up to 3 days.

SERVES 2

140g (just over 5oz) quinoa
360ml (12fl. oz) water
1 tsp Marigold Reduced Salt Vegetable Bouillon powder
3–4 tbsp fresh or frozen petit pois
2 tbsp cashew nuts
2 tsp sesame oil
1 tbsp tamari (wheat-free soy sauce, or use soy sauce)
2 tsp lemon juice
1 large carrot, julienned
6 spring onions, finely sliced on the diagonal
Freshly ground black pepper

1 Add the quinoa, water and bouillon powder to a saucepan and bring to the boil. Cover and simmer for around 13 minutes, or until all the water has been absorbed and the quinoa grains are soft and fluffy.
2 Add the peas and stir through, then remove from the heat. They will cook or soften slightly in the residual warmth.
3 Combine with all the other ingredients, tossing thoroughly to mix all the flavours and allow the quinoa to absorb the liquid seasonings.

GL PER SERVING: 6

COOK'S NOTES
SERVING SUGGESTION (PER PERSON) serve with a 4 GL starter or pudding to total 10 GL
VARIATIONS omit the cashews if you have a nut allergy – the quinoa provides complete protein on its own
ALLERGY SUITABILITY gluten, wheat, dairy free (use tamari instead of soy if you cannot eat wheat)

✓ MAINTENANCE PHASE
serve with a starter and/or pudding up to 9 GL to total 15 GL (such as 2 Almond pancakes (8 GL) (see page 172)

Lentil dahl

We both love this dahl. It's one of the easiest recipes in the book, yet is very moreish, low GL, and incredibly rich in antioxidants. We've doubled the recipe so you can freeze the remainder, or store in the fridge for up to 3 days.

SERVES 4

300g (11oz) red lentils, well rinsed and drained
600ml (1 pint) water
1 medium onion, chopped
4 cloves of garlic, crushed
4 tsp Marigold Reduced Salt Vegetable Bouillon powder
1 x 400g can chopped tomatoes
1 heaped tsp curry powder

1 Place the lentils in a saucepan with the water, onion, garlic and bouillon powder. Bring to the boil and simmer for 10 minutes before adding the tomatoes and curry powder and stirring well.
2 Cover and leave to simmer for a further 20 minutes, stirring occasionally to make sure it doesn't stick to the bottom of the pan. If it starts to get too thick, add a little water; if it seems too watery, leave uncovered. The lentils should form a porridge-like paste.

GL PER SERVING: 7

COOK'S NOTES
SERVING SUGGESTION (PER PERSON) serve with ½ wholemeal pitta bread or 35g quinoa (dry weight) to make a complete meal (total GL = 10.5)
ALLERGY SUITABILITY gluten, wheat, dairy, yeast free

✓ MAINTENANCE PHASE
serve with 45g (dry weight) brown basmati rice and a green salad (total GL = 15)

COOK'S NOTES

SERVING SUGGESTION (PER PERSON)
serve with 45g brown basmati rice (dry weight) (total GL= 9)

VARIATIONS use broccoli instead of cauliflower florets. If you like hot food, increase the quantity of cayenne pepper. Add chicken if you are not a vegetarian (fry it off first in a small amount of oil, then add it to the pan with the cauliflower to cook through)

ALLERGY SUITABILITY gluten, wheat, yeast free

MAINTENANCE PHASE
increase the brown basmati rice to 60g (dry weight) and have with a 3GL starter, drink or pudding (like Oriental chicken broth – see page 86) (total GL= 15)

Cauliflower dahl

A slightly more elaborate dahl. The addition of ginger and tumeric provides a spicier flavour and extra antioxidants. The al dente cauliflower – a superhealthy cruciferous vegetable rich in vitamins – provides bite and contrasts deliciously with the smooth lentils. You can double this recipe and freeze the remainder, or store in the fridge for up to 3 days.

SERVES 2

2 onions, diced
2 cloves of garlic, crushed
2cm (³/4 in) fresh root ginger, peeled and chopped (Tip: the easiest way to peel fresh ginger is to scrape off the skin with the edge of a teaspoon)
1/2 tsp turmeric
1/2 tsp ground cumin
1/4 tsp cayenne pepper
2 tsp coconut oil or olive oil
75g (3oz) split red lentils, well rinsed and drained
600ml (1pt) water
2 tsp Marigold Reduced Salt Vegetable Bouillon powder
1/3 medium-sized cauliflower, cut into small to medium-sized florets

1 Put the onions, garlic, ginger, turmeric, cumin and cayenne pepper into a blender and purée.
2 Heat the oil in a pan and add the puréed mixture, frying it over a medium heat for 5 minutes before adding the lentils, water and vegetable bouillon powder to the pan and boiling, uncovered, for 10 minutes.
3 Add the cauliflower, cover and simmer for 15 minutes, to allow the lentils to cook down to almost a purée and the cauliflower to soften.

Lentil stew

This thick, rich stew is ideal on colder nights. Red lentils are very low GL and contain phytoestrogens, which help balance hormones. As this recipe serves four, you can have it again the next day or freeze the remainder.

SERVES 4

1 tsp coconut oil or olive oil
1 clove of garlic, crushed
1 onion, chopped
1 green pepper, diced
1 small carrot, sliced
1 stick celery, sliced
125g (just under 5oz) red lentils, well rinsed and drained
2½ tsp Marigold Reduced Salt Vegetable Bouillon powder
180ml (6fl. oz) water
1 tsp dried mixed Italian herbs
12 cherry tomatoes, roughly chopped
1½ tbsp tomato purée
Freshly ground black pepper

1 Heat the oil in a large frying pan and add the garlic, cooking for 30 seconds or so before adding the onion. Sauté gently for 2 minutes.
2 Tip in the pepper, carrot and celery and cook for a further 5 minutes.
3 Add the lentils, bouillon powder, water and herbs to the pan and stir well. Allow the mixture to boil, uncovered, for 10 minutes.
4 Place the tomatoes and tomato purée in the pan, cover and reduce the heat, then simmer for a further 15 to 20 minutes or until the stew is thick and the lentils completely soft. Season with black pepper.

PER SERVING: 5

COOK'S NOTES
SERVING SUGGESTION (PER PERSON) serve with 40g wholemeal spaghetti (dry weight) or half a small baked potato or sweet potato (total GL = 12)
VARIATIONS use mushrooms in place of the celery or pepper. You could also use green lentils instead of red (cook according to pack instructions)
ALLERGY SUITABILITY gluten, wheat, dairy, yeast free

✓ MAINTENANCE PHASE
serve with 55g wholemeal spaghetti (dry weight) or 1 small baked potato or sweet potato (total GL = 15)

SERVING SUGGESTION (PER PERSON) serve with steamed cauliflower and peas (total GB = 9)

VARIATIONS use mushrooms in place of the celery or pepper in the Lentil stew

ALLERGY SUITABILITY gluten, wheat, dairy, yeast free

MAINTENANCE PHASE

serve with steamed cauliflower and peas, and either ½ a baked potato or a 6 GB starter or pudding to total 15 GB

Tip: to use up leftover egg yolks, store them in a covered container in the fridge for up to 2 days and add to scrambled eggs for breakfast (use one extra yolk per whole egg, adding them to the pan at the same time) for a rich breakfast packed with brain-boosting phospholipids.

Lentil moussaka with a soufflé crust

Fiona invented this recipe as a way of using up leftovers, but it is really excellent in its own right. The soufflé crust makes a delicious and unusual change from the standard cheese sauce topping.

SERVES 2

2 portions of Lentil stew (see page 137)
1 tbsp coconut oil or olive oil
1 small aubergine, sliced lengthways into about 6 slices
2 medium egg whites
100g (4oz) ready-made hummus

1 Preheat the oven to 190C/375F/Gas mark 5.
2 Make the Lentil stew as per the recipe instructions (see page 137).
3 Heat the oil in a large frying pan and gently fry the aubergine slices for around 2 minutes on each side until they turn golden and soften. Remove from the pan and set to one side to cool.
4 Beat the egg whites until they form stiff peaks. Using a metal spoon to prevent air escaping from the beaten egg, take one spoonful and fold gently into the hummus. Gradually fold the rest of the egg white into the hummus, taking care not to lose the air.
5 Place the lentil mixture into a small ovenproof dish, then arrange the aubergine slices on top, trying to cover the whole lentil mixture. Spoon the soufflé mixture on top carefully, then bake for 15 minutes until the topping is golden and slightly stiff to the touch.

Roasted pepper and artichoke tortilla

Spanish tortilla is a robust, colourful dish that can be enjoyed as a simple supper or on a picnic. While the potatoes in this recipe have a fairly high GL, the protein from the eggs balance out the overall GL score. This version uses antipasti vegetables, but you could use cooked leftover veg such as French beans, courgettes or mushrooms. Delicious hot or cold.

SERVES 2

150g (just over 5oz) baby new potatoes (around 8), scrubbed clean but not peeled, and cut into small cubes
1 tbsp coconut oil or olive oil
2 cloves of garlic, crushed
150g (just over 5oz) or 2 roasted red peppers, either from the deli or a jar or roasted at home (see recipe on page 126), cubed
2 tbsp marinated artichoke hearts, drained and mashed or chopped into chunks
4 medium eggs
Freshly ground black pepper
Low-sodium salt or sea salt
1/2 tsp dried oregano

1 Place the potatoes in a small pan and just cover with cold water. Bring to the boil and simmer, covered, for around 10 minutes, or until the potatoes are soft. Drain and set to one side.
2 Heat the oil in a medium-sized frying pan (use a small pan if you are halving the quantities to make a tortilla for one person) and fry the garlic for 30 seconds. Add the potatoes and sauté for 5 minutes or so.
3 Stir the peppers and artichokes into the pan and reduce the heat.
4 Beat the eggs with the pepper, a little salt and the oregano. Pour evenly over the vegetable mixture in the pan and stir to expose the egg on top to the heat on the base of the pan. Leave the tortilla cooking over a low-medium heat for around 6 minutes or until the eggs are set (the edges and base should be set, with the top still a little soft as it carries on cooking after you remove it from the heat).
5 Remove the pan from the heat and loosen the edges and base with a palette knife. Turn the tortilla out onto a plate. Serve hot or cold.

PER SERVING: 11

COOK'S NOTES
SERVING SUGGESTION (PER PERSON) serve with a mixed leaf salad (total GL = 11)
VARIATIONS omit the artichokes if preferred, and use double the amount of peppers, or add some pitted black olives or sun blush tomatoes
ALLERGY SUITABILITY gluten, wheat, dairy free

MAINTENANCE PHASE
serve with a 4 GL starter or pudding to total 15 GL

Teriyaki tofu

In this simple dish the fabulous flavour of Japanese Teriyaki sauce transforms plain tofu.

GL PER SERVING: 4

COOK'S NOTES
SERVING SUGGESTION (PER PERSON) serve with 45g brown basmati rice (dry weight) and a small amount of steamed or steam-fried vegetables (such as beansprouts, spring onions, mangetout or peppers) (total GL = 12)
ALLERGY SUITABILITY gluten, wheat, dairy free

✓ MAINTENANCE PHASE
increase the brown basmati rice to 60g (dry weight) and serve with the vegetables as above (total GL = 16)

SERVES 2

1 x 250g (9oz) pack plain organic tofu (Cauldron Foods tofu is readily available in supermarkets), patted dry with kitchen towel and cubed
2 portions of Teriyaki sauce (see page 157)
1 tbsp coconut oil or olive oil

1 Marinate the tofu in the Teriyaki sauce in the fridge for 30 minutes if you have time (don't worry if you don't, it will still work but simply won't have the same depth of flavour).
2 Heat the oil in a large frying pan. Using a slotted spoon, take the tofu out of the marinade, reserving this for later. Stir-fry the tofu on all sides.
3 When the tofu starts to turn a pale golden colour, remove it from the heat and pour the reserved marinade into the pan. Return to the heat for a few seconds to thicken, then serve.

Marinated tofu couscous

A ridiculously easy meal – the couscous cooks in 4 minutes flat and the tofu pieces are simply stirred in. Lemon, herbs and fresh veg add extra flavour and bite. Ideal for an impromptu al fresco lunch or to take to work.

GL PER SERVING: 12

COOK'S NOTES
VARIATIONS replace the couscous with quinoa for a gluten-free version that is only 7 GL
ALLERGY SUITABILITY dairy free

✓ MAINTENANCE PHASE
serve with a 3 GL starter, pudding or drink (such as St Clement's smoothie – see page 182) to total GL 15

SERVES 2

100g (4oz) Belazu barley couscous (or just use standard wheat couscous)
1½ tsp Marigold Reduced Salt Vegetable Bouillon powder
1 x 150g pack Cauldron Foods Golden Marinated Tofu Pieces (from the chiller cabinet in supermarkets)
2 tsp lemon juice
5 spring onions, finely chopped on the diagonal
6 cherry tomatoes, thinly sliced
½ tbsp fresh flat leaf parsley leaves, finely chopped

1 Cook the couscous by placing it in a bowl and adding enough boiling water to just cover it. Add the bouillon powder and cover with a clean tea towel for 4 minutes to allow it to soften and absorb the water.
2 When the couscous is ready, stir it through with a fork to break up the grains, then mix in the rest of the ingredients.

Halloumi and aubergine curry

An unusual curry that's super-quick to make. Halloumi works very well pan-fried, as it holds its shape even when heated and becomes wonderfully squidgy inside.

SERVES 2

1 heaped tsp medium-strength curry powder
200g (7oz) halloumi cheese, cubed into pieces about 1cm (1/2in) square
1 tsp coconut oil or olive oil
2 cloves of garlic, crushed
1 aubergine, cubed into pieces about 1cm (1/2in) square

1 Sprinkle the curry powder over the halloumi cubes and stir them to coat well.
2 Heat the oil in a large frying pan and cook the garlic for 30 seconds before adding the halloumi pieces. Cook for a couple of minutes.
3 Add the aubergine to the pan and continue sautéing the curry for another 8 minutes or so, until the aubergine softens and colours, stirring from time to time to cook the halloumi cubes on all sides.

GL PER SERVING: 2

COOK'S NOTES
SERVING SUGGESTION (PER PERSON) serve with 45g brown basmati rice (dry weight) and salad (total GL = 10)
ALLERGY SUITABILITY gluten, wheat free

✓ **MAINTENANCE PHASE**
increase the brown basmati rice to 60g (dry weight) and salad (total GL = 13)

Halloumi kebabs

Halloumi is perfect for kebabs because it holds its shape when heated. This recipe, which uses fajita spices, combines the Cypriot cheese with vitamin-packed veg. It's a good party dish, as the kebabs can be made in advance.

SERVES 2

2 tbsp fajita spices (from a packet)
1 tbsp olive oil
200g (7oz) halloumi cheese, cut into bite-sized cubes
1 red or orange pepper, cut into similar sized squares as the halloumi
1 courgette, cut into bite-sized chunks
6 cherry tomatoes, whole

1 Preheat the oven to 190C/375F/Gas mark 5 and soak 4 wooden skewers in a bowl of water for at least 5 minutes to stop the wood from splitting in the oven. Alternatively, use metal skewers, which don't require pre-soaking.
2 Tip the spices and oil into a bowl and mix to form a paste.
3 Add the halloumi and vegetable chunks to the bowl and stir to coat evenly in the paste.
4 Spear the chunks evenly on the 4 skewers and place on a baking tray.
5 Bake for 12 to 15 minutes.

GL PER SERVING: 4

COOK'S NOTES
SERVING SUGGESTION (PER PERSON) serve with 70g quinoa (dry weight) or 45g brown basmati rice (dry weight) (total GL = 11)
VARIATIONS use mushrooms instead of the cherry tomatoes or courgette
ALLERGY SUITABILITY gluten, wheat free (make sure you choose gluten-free fajita spices if necessary)

✓ **MAINTENANCE PHASE**
serve in 1 wrap with lettuce for a vegetarian fajita or with 60g brown basmati rice (dry weight) and salad (total GL = 15)

PESTOS

With its beneficial oils, antioxidant-rich herbs and punchy flavours, a dollop of pesto adds life to all kinds of food – pasta or beans, baked potatoes, soups, and chicken or fish fillets. Here we've come up with combinations that are just as delicious as basil with pine nuts, but more inventive and interesting – and every bit as good without the Parmesan. Note that for all the pesto recipes, you can quadruple the recipe and store in the fridge for up to 4 days.

GL PER SERVING: 2

COOK'S NOTES
SERVING SUGGESTION (PER PERSON) with 55g wholemeal pasta or spaghetti (dry weight) and salad (total GL = 12)
ALLERGY SUITABILITY gluten, wheat, dairy free

MAINTENANCE PHASE double up the pesto quantities (to make 2 tablespoons per person) and serve with 55g wholemeal pasta or spaghetti (dry weight) and salad (total GL = 14)

Sun-dried tomato and black olive pesto

The intense flavours of sun-dried tomatoes and olives are delicious with wholemeal pasta or mixed with chickpeas or borlotti beans and chopped fresh vegetables for a quick, substantial salad.

SERVES 2 (MAKES 2 TABLESPOONS OF PESTO)
50g (2oz) sun-dried tomato paste (available in jars or tubes from supermarkets)
50g (2oz) black olives, pitted
50g (2oz) pine nuts
10g (just under $1/2$ oz) flat leaf parsley leaves
25g (1oz) basil leaves
2 cloves of garlic, crushed
1 dsp lemon juice
1 tbsp olive oil
Freshly ground black pepper

Place all of the ingredients in a small food processor or mini chopper and blend until fairly smooth.

Pumpkin seed pesto

It's wonderful when something that tastes this amazing is also really good for you – pumpkin seed butter and Essential Balance Oil are both rich in omega-3s. Stir this dark-green pesto through soup or pasta, spread on rye bread or add to bean or lentil salads.

SERVES 2 (MAKES 2 TABLESPOONS OF PESTO)
25g (1oz) pumpkin seeds
40g (1½ oz) pumpkin seed butter (available from
  Health Products for Life) see page 187
10g (just under ½ oz) flat leaf parsley leaves
10g (just under ½ oz) basil leaves
1 clove of garlic, crushed
½ dsp lemon juice
½ tbsp Essential Balance Oil (available from Health
  Products for Life) or olive oil

1 Grind the pumpkin seeds until roughly chopped.
2 Place the pumpkin seed butter in a small blender or food processor with the pumpkin seeds, herbs, garlic and lemon juice. Blitz until the mixture is well combined.
3 Add the oil and mix until the pesto is an even consistency.

(GL) PER SERVING: 1

COOK'S NOTES
SERVING SUGGESTION (PER PERSON)
with 55g wholemeal pasta or spaghetti (dry weight) and salad (total (GL) = 11)
ALLERGY SUITABILITY gluten, wheat, dairy, yeast free

✓ MAINTENANCE PHASE
double up the pesto quantities (to make 2 tablespoons per person) and serve with 55g wholemeal pasta or spaghetti (dry weight) and salad (total (GL) = 13)

Feta and roast pepper pesto

There's a zesty mix of flavours in this pesto from the feta, pine nuts and sweet roasted peppers – which also give it its beautiful orange colour.

SERVES 2 (MAKES 2 TABLESPOONS OF PESTO)
50g (2oz) roasted red peppers, from the deli
  or a jar or roasted at home (see page 126)
50g (2oz) pine nuts
50g (2oz) feta cheese
Freshly ground black pepper
2 cloves of garlic, crushed

Place all the ingredients in a small food processor or mini chopper and blend until fairly smooth.

(GL) PER SERVING: 1

COOK'S NOTES
SERVING SUGGESTION (PER PERSON)
serve with 55g wholemeal pasta or spaghetti (dry weight) and salad (total (GL) = 11)
ALLERGY SUITABILITY gluten, wheat free

✓ MAINTENANCE PHASE
double up the pesto quantities (to make 2 tablespoons per person) and serve with 55g wholemeal pasta or spaghetti (dry weight) and salad (total (GL) = 13)

Walnut and goat's cheese pesto

The walnuts in this delicious pesto provide adequate oil, so you don't need to add extra. Even better, walnut oil contains omega-3s, which are vital for the health of skin, heart and brain.

SERVES 2 (MAKES 2 TABLESPOONS OF PESTO)
50g (2oz) mild, soft goat's cheese
50g (2oz) chopped walnuts
25g (1oz) fresh basil
1 dsp of lemon juice
Freshly ground black pepper
1 clove of garlic, crushed

Place all the ingredients in a small food processor or mini chopper and blend until fairly smooth.

(GL) PER SERVING: 1

COOK'S NOTES
SERVING SUGGESTION (PER PERSON)
serve with 55g wholemeal pasta or spaghetti (dry weight) and salad (total (GL) = 11)
VARIATIONS use 50g (2oz) pine nuts instead of the walnuts and add 50g (2oz) pitted Kalamata olives
ALLERGY SUITABILITY gluten, wheat free

✓ MAINTENANCE PHASE
double up the pesto quantities (to make 2 tablespoons per person) and serve with 55g wholemeal pasta or spaghetti (dry weight) and salad (total (GL) = 13)

Aubergine pâté

The aubergine and borlotti beans give a smoky flavour to this delicious pâté, which is also rich in antioxidants from the onion, garlic and tomato purée. You can double this recipe and store in the fridge for up to 3 days.

SERVES 2
1 tsp coconut oil or olive oil
1 clove of garlic, crushed
1 red onion, diced
1/4 medium aubergine, cubed
1 tbsp tomato purée
1/2 can borlotti beans, rinsed and drained
1/2 tsp mixed dried herbs
1 tsp Marigold Reduced Salt Vegetable Bouillon powder
Freshly ground black pepper

1 Heat the oil and sauté the garlic for 30 seconds or so before adding the onion and cooking till it softens.
2 Throw in the aubergine and cook for a few minutes until it browns and softens.
3 Stir in the tomato purée, beans, dried herbs and bouillon powder and stir together, then season with black pepper.
4 Place the mixture in a food processor and blitz until it is fairly smooth.

(GL) PER SERVING: 5

COOK'S NOTES
SERVING SUGGESTION (PER PERSON)
serve on 1 slice of toasted, thin pumpkernickel style rye bread with some rocket (total (GL) = 10)
ALLERGY SUITABILITY gluten, wheat, dairy, yeast free

✓ MAINTENANCE PHASE
serve with 2 thin slices pumpernickel style rye bread and rocket (total (GL) = 15)

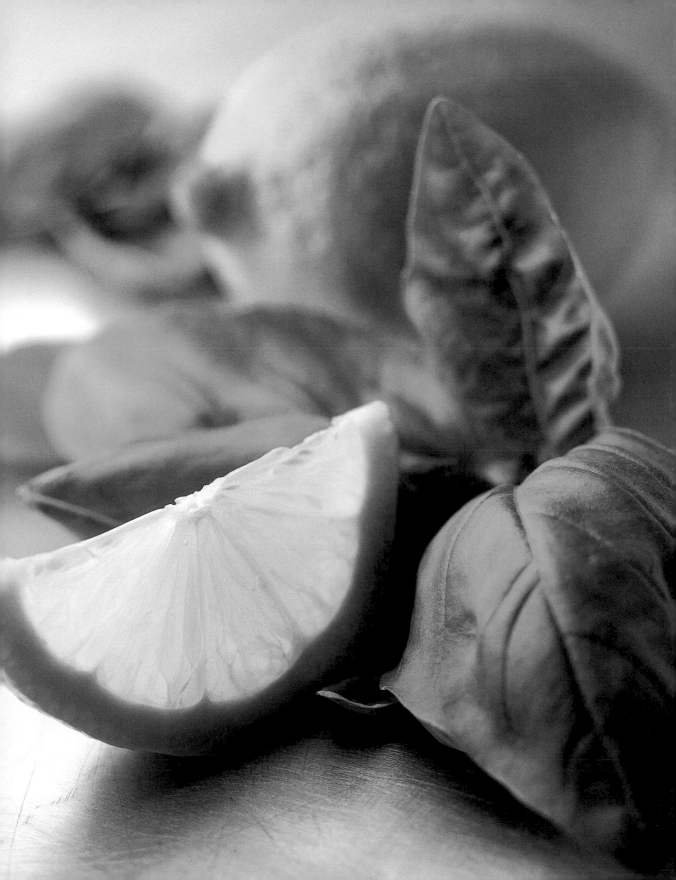

ACCOMPANIMENTS

Side dishes can make a meal, providing extra flavour and nutrients.

We've designed this cookbook so that you can mix and match main meals and accompaniments and still meet your GL limits per meal – just check the GL scores for each. Bear in mind that these side dishes also make brilliant partners for plain and simple grilled fish, chicken or smoked tofu. You're certainly spoilt for choice, with Cashew cauliflower cheese, Roast butternut squash with shallots, Spicy cherry tomato potato salad, and a range of delicious sauces, all packed with flavour and phytonutrients to keep your meals balanced and ever-interesting.

Remember: You should aim to eat 10 GL both at lunch and at dinner to lose weight, and 15 GL once you have reached the maintenance phase. You can use recipes from the accompaniments section when you need to add extra GL to reach your main meal GL score.

And of course, if you'd rather create your own accompaniments, you can choose from all the non-starchy veg described in Part 1 on page 23 and the table on page 90.

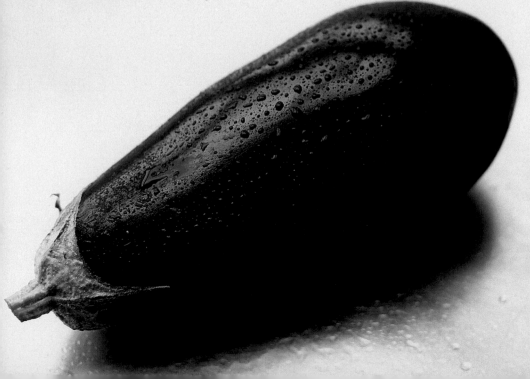

Steamed Savoy cabbage with crème fraîche

With its dark green leaves, mild taste and superior nutritive content, Savoy cabbage makes a welcome change from the ordinary white kind. This dish is smart enough for a dinner party.

SERVES 2
1/2 a Savoy cabbage (approximately 200g/7oz), outer leaves removed and the rest rinsed, dried and thinly sliced
3 tbsp crème fraîche
1/2 tbsp fresh flat leaf parsley leaves, finely chopped
Pinch of low-sodium salt or sea salt
Freshly ground black pepper

1 Steam the cabbage for 6 minutes, then remove from the heat and place in a pan.
2 Stir the crème fraîche and parsley into the cabbage, allowing the crème fraîche to melt in the heat from the cabbage, and season with salt and pepper.

PER SERVING: 2

COOK'S NOTES
SERVING SUGGESTION (PER PERSON)
serve with chicken or fish – it's particularly delicious with smoked fish
ALLERGY SUITABILITY gluten, wheat free

Cashew cauliflower cheese

The sauce for this scrumptious recipe thickens up brilliantly thanks to the ground cashews and sunflower seeds, and can be made without Parmesan if you're avoiding dairy products.

SERVES 2
1/2 large cauliflower, cut into florets
1 tsp Marigold Reduced Salt Vegetable Bouillon powder
25g (1oz) cashew nuts, finely ground
25g (1oz) sunflower seeds, finely ground
90ml (3fl oz) water
1 tbsp cornflour
Freshly ground black pepper
150ml (1/4 pt) skimmed milk, soya milk or nut milk
Large pinch of grated nutmeg
25g (1oz) Parmesan shavings (optional)

1 Preheat the oven to 200C/400F/Gas mark 6.
2 Steam the cauliflower florets for around 15 to 20 minutes, until just tender when pierced with a knife.
3 Meanwhile, start on the sauce by mixing the bouillon powder, ground cashews and sunflower seeds, water, cornflour and pepper in a pan and bring to the boil. (Don't be alarmed when it thickens rapidly to form a lump.) Simmer gently as you gradually add the milk (as you would for a standard white sauce recipe), stirring to make a thick, smooth sauce.
4 Place the cauliflower in a shallow ovenproof dish and pour the sauce over the top. Sprinkle with nutmeg and either serve immediately or top with the Parmesan shavings (if using) and bake for 20 minutes until the cheese is melted, or grill for around 5 minutes until the cheese melts and bubbles.

PER SERVING: 3

COOK'S NOTES
SERVING SUGGESTION (PER PERSON)
serve with chicken or fish and potatoes
VARIATIONS use broccoli instead of cauliflower
ALLERGY SUITABILITY gluten, wheat free

Lemon and mint petits pois

Mint and citrus lend an extra zing to the flavour of peas. Frozen petits pois work just as well as fresh peas and are super-convenient – plus they won't have lost their nutrients under supermarket striplighting.

SERVES 2

150g (just over 5oz) frozen petits pois (if using fresh peas in the pod you will need twice this weight, and to shell them)
1 tbsp olive oil
1 tbsp lemon juice
3 tbsp fresh mint, finely chopped
Freshly ground black pepper, to taste
Pinch of low-sodium salt or sea salt

1 Put the peas in a small saucepan and just cover with boiling water.
2 Cover and simmer for 3 minutes, then drain any remaining water, toss with the oil, lemon juice and mint and season.

PER SERVING: 3

COOK'S NOTES
SERVING SUGGESTION (PER PERSON)
serve with fish or chicken and other cooked vegetables, or toss through a salad
ALLERGY SUITABILITY gluten, wheat, dairy, yeast free

Baked fennel

Slow-roasting fennel brings out its wonderful sweetness and softens the aniseed flavour. Absolutely fantastic with fish.

SERVES 2

2 fennel bulbs
2 dsp of lemon juice
2 tbsp olive oil
Pinch of low-sodium salt or sea salt
Freshly ground black pepper

1 Preheat the oven to 200C/400F/Gas mark 6.
2 Trim the roots from the fennel, remove the outer leaves and slice lengthways into quarters.
3 Place in a roasting tin and sprinkle with the lemon juice, oil and seasoning. Cover the tin with tin foil and bake for 45 minutes, until soft.

PER SERVING: 3

COOK'S NOTES
SERVING SUGGESTION (PER PERSON)
serve with fish or meat, or quinoa for vegetarians
ALLERGY SUITABILITY gluten, wheat, dairy, yeast free

Roasted vegetables

A deservedly popular way of cooking vegetables. Using lots of differently coloured veg will give you a variety of nutrients and mingled flavours, and it can all be done in one roasting tin.

SERVES 2
4 shallots, peeled, whole
10 cherry tomatoes, whole
10 button or small mushrooms, cleaned with a brush
  or wiped with kitchen towel and left whole
1 courgette, cut into chunks
$1/2$ aubergine, cut into chunks
2 tbsp olive oil

1 Preheat the oven to 190C/375F/Gas mark 5.
2 Place the vegetables in a roasting tin and drizzle with the olive oil, mixing them around to coat thoroughly.
3 Bake for 25 minutes.

Cannellini bean mash

This beany mash is much lower in GLs than the ubiquitous potato type, and full of great flavours and hormone-balancing phytonutrients. Served with fish or meat, it's delicious warm but can even be served cold. You can double this recipe and store in the fridge for up to 3 days.

SERVES 2
1 x 410g can cannellini beans, rinsed and drained
1 tbsp skimmed milk, soya milk or nut milk
1 tsp Marigold Reduced Salt Vegetable Bouillon powder
1 tbsp olive oil
Freshly ground black pepper

1 Purée the beans roughly using a blender.
2 Place in a pan with the rest of the ingredients and heat through, mashing until fairly smooth.

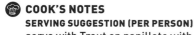

Avocado potato salad

You won't miss mayonnaise with this salad – mashed avocado is just as creamy, but contains far healthier fats and tastes delicious mixed in with baby new potatoes.

SERVES 2

100g (4oz) baby new potatoes, scrubbed clean
1/2 tsp Marigold Reduced Salt Vegetable Bouillon powder
1/2 ripe avocado, mashed with a fork with 1 tbsp lemon juice
1/2 tbsp fresh flat leaf parsley leaves, chopped
Freshly ground black pepper

1 Boil the potatoes in water with the bouillon powder for 30 minutes, or until soft. Drain.
2 When the potatoes have cooled, stir in the mashed avocado and sprinkle with parsley and black pepper.

GL PER SERVING: 5

COOK'S NOTES
SERVING SUGGESTION (PER PERSON) serve with chicken or Nick's beefburgers (see page 97) (total GL = 16)
ALLERGY SUITABILITY gluten, wheat, dairy, yeast free

Spicy cherry tomato potato salad

This fiery, Spanish-inspired potato salad is best served warm, and would be perfect for a summer meal paired with plain grilled chicken or fish.

SERVES 2

100g (4oz) baby new potatoes, scrubbed clean
1/4 tsp Marigold Reduced Salt Vegetable Bouillon powder
1/2 tbsp coconut oil or olive oil
1 clove of garlic, crushed
1/4 mild red chilli, deseeded and finely chopped
1/2 good tsp paprika
30ml (1fl. oz) tomato passata
1/2 good handful cherry tomatoes, halved
1/2 tsp xylitol
Freshly ground black pepper
1/2 tbsp fresh flat leaf parsley leaves, chopped
2 spring onions, sliced on the diagonal

1 Boil the potatoes in water with the bouillon powder for 30 minutes, or until soft.
2 While the potatoes are cooking, heat the oil in a pan and gently fry the garlic, chilli and paprika for a couple of minutes.
3 Add the passata, the cherry tomatoes and the xylitol and simmer for around 10 minutes.
4 Drain the potatoes, return to their saucepan and pour in the tomato sauce. Season with black pepper and sprinkle with parsley and spring onions and mix it all together. Serve warm.

GL PER SERVING: 6

COOK'S NOTES
SERVING SUGGESTION (PER PERSON) serve with chicken or fish and salad
ALLERGY SUITABILITY gluten, wheat, dairy, yeast free

Puy lentils

Puy lentils hold their shape when cooked, so they retain a bit
of bite along with their wonderful earthy flavour. Keep a packet
in your larder for a quick low-GL staple that goes brilliantly
with meat, fish or rice.

SERVES 2
225g (8oz) Puy lentils, well rinsed and drained
4 tsp Marigold Reduced Salt Vegetable Bouillon powder
Freshly ground black pepper

1 Place the Puy lentils in a pan and add enough water to cover
them, plus the bouillon powder.
2 Bring to the boil, cover and simmer for 15 to 20 minutes until
the lentils are tender to the bite and the water is absorbed.

Sweet potato wedges

A moreish yet much healthier alternative to chips, these
wedges are baked instead of fried. Sweet potatoes are very
good for the immune system – the orange flesh contains
the antioxidant betacarotene.

SERVES 2
1 medium sweet potato, washed but unpeeled, cut into wedges
1/2 tbsp olive oil

1 Preheat the oven to 180C/350F/Gas mark 4.
2 Place the wedges on a baking tray and drizzle with the oil,
shaking to coat, then bake for 40 minutes, turning the wedges
halfway through cooking.

Roast butternut squash with shallots

This great partnering of butternut squash and shallots cooks down to a wonderful melt-in-the-mouth squidginess. Like all orange fruit and vegetables, the squash is a good source of betacarotene, too, which your body converts to vitamin A.

SERVES 2

1/2 small butternut squash (approximately 325g/just under 12oz pre-prepared weight), peeled, deseeded and cut into bite-sized chunks
8 shallots, peeled
1 tbsp olive oil
Freshly ground black pepper

1 Preheat the oven to 200C/400F/Gas mark 6.
2 Place the squash and shallots in a roasting tin and drizzle with oil, shaking them around to coat evenly.
3 Put in the oven and cook for around an hour, shaking the tray again half way through.
4 When the squash is fairly soft when pierced with a knife, remove from the oven and season with black pepper.

PER SERVING: 8

COOK'S NOTES
SERVING SUGGESTION (PER PERSON)
serve with Hot smoked salmon with crème fraîche and herb sauce (see page 109) (total = 10)
ALLERGY SUITABILITY gluten, wheat, dairy, yeast free

Giant baked beans

'Giant' beans are a classic Greek meze, or snack. They're simply plump butterbeans in a rich tomato and herb sauce – miles better than sugary baked beans. Try these with organic sausages. You can double this recipe and freeze the remainder, or store in the fridge for up to 3 days.

SERVES 2

1 onion, finely chopped
2 tsp coconut oil or olive oil
1 x 410g can butterbeans, rinsed and drained
2 tbsp tomato purée
1 x 200g can chopped tomatoes
1 1/2 tsp Marigold Reduced Salt Vegetable Bouillon powder
1/2 tsp herbes de Provence

1 Sauté the onion in the oil until transparent.
2 Stir in the rest of the ingredients and simmer for a couple of minutes until combined.

PER SERVING: 8

COOK'S NOTES
SERVING SUGGESTION (PER PERSON)
serve with a cooked chicken breast or 2 lean, good-quality sausages (total = 10)
ALLERGY SUITABILITY gluten, wheat, dairy, yeast free

MAINTENANCE PHASE
serve on 1 medium slice wholemeal toast (total = 15)

Sweet potato and carrot mash

A beautiful orangey mash rich in flavour and betacarotene, this is far more sophisticated than mashed potato but just as satisfying. Leaving the sweet potatoes unpeeled preserves more nutrients and fibre, but you could peel them if you prefer. You can double this recipe and store in the fridge for up to 3 days.

SERVES 2

1 medium sweet potato, unpeeled
1 medium carrot
1/2 tsp Marigold Reduced Salt Vegetable Bouillon powder
Freshly ground black pepper

1 Slice the sweet potato and carrot thinly and steam for around 12 minutes until soft.
2 Place in a pan and mash roughly, then stir in the seasoning and warm through.

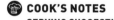
Flageolet beans in white sauce

The delicate flavour of flageolet beans is often unfairly overlooked in favour of more robust varieties such as kidney beans. In France they are rightly very popular. Here, they are delicious with the creamy white sauce. You can double this recipe and store in the fridge for up to 3 days.

SERVES 2

1 x 410g can flageolet beans, rinsed and drained
2 portions of Tahini white sauce (see page 156)

Make the sauce according to the recipe instructions, then stir the beans into the sauce in a pan and heat gently.

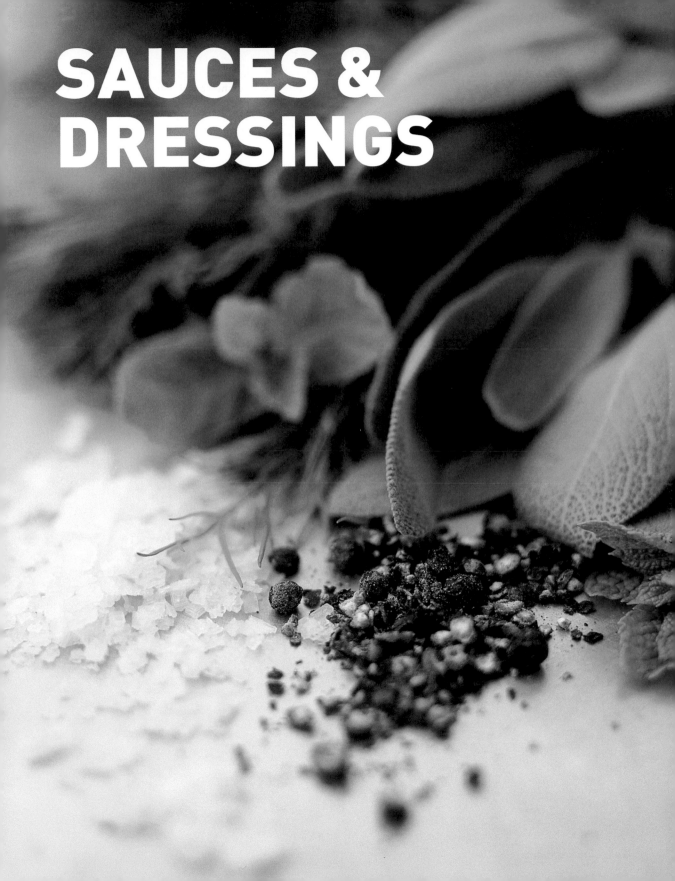

SAUCES & DRESSINGS

Crème fraîche and herb sauce

Made in seconds, this elegant sauce will make your guests think you have been slaving over a hot stove for far longer. It's mild and tangy and goes very well with all kinds of dishes, from grains to fish.

SERVES 2
2 tbsp low-fat crème fraîche
1 tbsp fresh flat leaf parsley leaves, finely chopped
Pinch of low-sodium salt or sea salt
Freshly ground black pepper to taste

Gently melt the crème fraîche and stir in the herbs. Season to taste.

PER SERVING: 1

COOK'S NOTES
SERVING SUGGESTION (PER PERSON)
pour over fish, poultry, grain or vegetable dishes
ALLERGY SUITABILITY gluten, wheat free

Tahini white sauce

The tahini and vegetable bouillon powder in this recipe impart a wonderful full-bodied flavour to this cheeseless white sauce. If avoiding dairy, use soya milk or a nut milk.

SERVES 2
210ml (7fl oz) skimmed milk, soya milk or nut milk
1 tbsp cornflour
1 tbsp tahini
2 tsp Marigold Reduced Salt Vegetable Bouillon powder

1 Stir half of the milk into the cornflour and mix until smooth.
2 Place in a pan with the tahini and bouillon powder and stir constantly over a gentle heat for around 3 to 5 minutes, gradually adding the rest of the milk to make a smooth, thick sauce.

PER SERVING: 4

COOK'S NOTES
SERVING SUGGESTION (PER PERSON)
serve with chicken or fish, or over bean or vegetable dishes
ALLERGY SUITABILITY gluten, wheat, dairy, yeast free

Teriyaki sauce

A wonderfully versatile sauce from Japan, adding instant depth of flavour to meat, fish, tofu and vegetables. You can double this recipe and store in the fridge for up to 3 days.

SERVES 2

1 tbsp tamari (wheat-free soy sauce) or soy sauce
1 tbsp mirin (Japanese rice cooking wine)
2 tsp grated fresh root ginger (Tip: the easiest way to peel fresh ginger is to scrape the skin off using the edge of a teaspoon)
1/2 tsp xylitol

Mix all of the ingredients together.

PER SERVING: 1

COOK'S NOTES
SERVING SUGGESTION (PER PERSON) use as a marinade for meat, fish or tofu, or simply as a dipping sauce or sauce for stir-fries or steam-fries
ALLERGY SUITABILITY gluten, wheat, dairy free

Tahini dressing

If you love mayonnaise, try this tahini dressing. It gives you the same creamy, emollient texture, but has a punchier taste and contains beneficial fats from the sesame tahini and olive oil as well as plenty of antioxidant nutrients. You can double this recipe and store in the fridge for up to 3 days.

SERVES 2

1 tbsp tahini
1 clove of garlic, crushed
2 tbsp olive oil
1 tsp sesame oil
1 tsp fresh flat leaf parsley leaves, finely chopped
1/2 tsp ground cumin
1 dsp lemon juice
Freshly ground black pepper

Mix all of the ingredients together until smooth.

PER SERVING: 1

COOK'S NOTES
SERVING SUGGESTION (PER PERSON) good with salad or crudités or as a dipping sauce for the Greek salad skewers (see page 78)(total = 6)
VARIATIONS adjust the seasoning according to taste
ALLERGY SUITABILITY gluten, wheat, dairy, yeast free

Oriental dressing

This will give flavour to steam-fries, stir-fries and fresh soba noodles. Fresh ginger is extremely good for you as it has strong anti-viral and anti-inflammatory properties. It also contains zinc, which is essential for immune function, so it is a good idea to include it in your diet as much as possible.

PER SERVING: 1

COOK'S NOTES
SERVING SUGGESTION (PER PERSON) lovely over fish, meat, tofu and vegetables
ALLERGY SUITABILITY gluten, wheat, dairy free

SERVES 2
2 tsp sesame oil
2 tbsp tamari (wheat-free soy sauce) or soy sauce
2 tsp fresh root ginger, peeled and finely chopped (Tip: the easiest way to peel fresh ginger is to scrape the skin off with the edge of a teaspoon)
2 cloves of garlic, crushed
2 tsp Mirin (Japanese rice cooking wine – available in the Oriental section of good supermarkets or food stores)
4 tbsp cold water

Mix all the ingredients together.

Lemon and garlic dressing

This simple dressing with the classic Mediterranean flavours of lemon and garlic makes green salads much more interesting. Garlic is very good for the immune system and should be eaten regularly – you will just have to apologise to anyone sitting near you! You can double this recipe and store in the fridge for up to 3 days.

PER SERVING: 1

COOK'S NOTES
ALLERGY SUITABILITY gluten, wheat, dairy, yeast free

SERVES 2
4 tbsp extra virgin olive oil
1 tbsp lemon juice
1 tsp Dijon mustard
1 clove of garlic, crushed
Freshly ground black pepper
Pinch of low-sodium salt or sea salt
Pinch of xylitol or caster sugar
Good pinch of paprika
Good pinch of curry powder
Good pinch of dried herbes de Provence

Mix all the ingredients together and adjust seasoning according to taste.

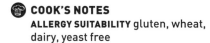

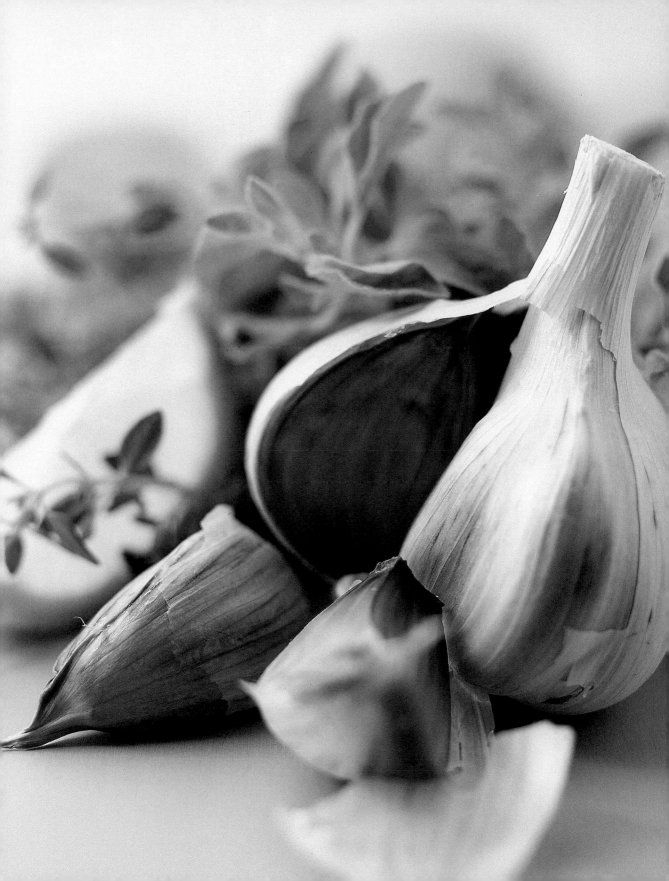

SWEET SNACKS & PUDDINGS

No self-respecting cookbook should be without a chapter on puddings! We just don't see the point of depriving yourself of delicious food, and that includes sweets. In any case, we're firmly convinced that the odd treat helps you stick to a healthy eating programme. And you'll find plenty of mouthwatering ones here, from 5GL biscuits and cakes for tea-time or elevenses, to higher GL puddings for special occasions once you've reached the maintenance phase.

These recipes would impress anyone, not just dieters grateful for anything that isn't green, and they manage it even though they're sugar-free and full of nutrients. They get their sweetness from the low-carb sugar alternative xylitol, and from nutritious fruits, nuts and seeds.

There's just one word of advice we'd like to give you. Please resist the higher GL puddings until you have been following the weight-loss plan for three weeks, and then have them about once a week until you reach the maintenance phase. There are lots of other fantastic choices in the meantime, including plenty of scrumptious fruit and yoghurt-based desserts.

Remember: aim to eat 5 GL for both your mid-morning and mid-afternoon snacks to lose weight, and the same once you have reached the maintenance phase.

See Part 1 pages 20–1 for a list of fruit that you can snack on for 5 GL

Your drinks and/or pudding allowance is 5 GL in total for weight loss and 10 GL for maintenance.

(cook) **COOK'S NOTES**

SERVING SUGGESTION (PER PERSON)
have this as a special occasion treat
only when you have reached the
maintenance phase. As it is 1GL
point above the allowance for
puddings and drinks, make sure the
main course preceding it comes in
at 14 (GL) or under.
ALLERGY SUITABILITY gluten, wheat,
dairy, yeast free (check that the
chocolate is dairy free)

**HEALTH NOTE: BECAUSE THIS
RECIPE CONTAINS RAW EGG,
ALWAYS CHOOSE ORGANIC OR AT
THE VERY LEAST FREE RANGE
EGGS TO REDUCE THE
LIKELIHOOD OF SALMONELLA
CONTAMINATION, AND DO NOT
SERVE TO PREGNANT WOMEN,
YOUNG CHILDREN, THE ELDERLY
OR INFIRM.**

Chocolate hazelnut mousse

Did you ever eat chocolate spread straight off the spoon as a
child? If so, you'll adore this nutty, moreish mousse. The nuts
also provide extra protein, which helps to lower the (GL). Steer
clear of cheap chocolate, which often uses harmful hydrogenated
fats instead of cocoa butter. You can double this recipe and store
in the fridge for up to 3 days.

SERVES 2
75g (3oz) good quality dark chocolate (around 70 per cent
    cocoa solids), broken into pieces
50g (2oz) hazelnuts, ground
2 organic, free range eggs, separated

1 Gently melt the chocolate. To do this, half-fill a saucepan with
water and let simmer. Place the chocolate in a small metal or heat-
proof bowl that fits the rim of the saucepan but does not touch the
water, and allow it to melt over the heat, stirring occasionally.
2 Remove the bowl from the heat and briskly stir the ground nuts
and egg yolks (one at a time) into the chocolate.
3 Beat the egg whites until they form stiff peaks. Using a metal
spoon to prevent air escaping from the beaten egg, take one spoonful
and fold gently into the chocolate mixture. Gradually fold the rest
of the egg white into the mixture, taking care not to lose the air.
4 Carefully spoon the mousse into 2 ramekins or into a bowl and
place in the fridge to set (this will take at least an hour).

Baked chocolate orange pots

This scrummy pudding is a cross between a mousse and a brownie. The outside and top form a sponge while the centre remains wonderfully gooey. The recipe serves 4 (it's pretty hard to split an egg in half to make it serve 2) so it's ideal for pudding when you've got friends over for dinner.

SERVES 4

1/2 tsp cornflour
3/4 tsp cocoa powder
20g (just under 1 oz) xylitol
50ml (just under 2fl. oz) skimmed milk, soya milk or nut milk
Juice of 1/2 a medium orange
1 large egg, separated
25g (1oz) good quality dark chocolate (around 70 per cent) cocoa solids), broken into fairly small pieces

1 Preheat the oven to 180C/350F/Gas mark 4.
2 Add the cornflour, cocoa and xylitol to a saucepan and gradually stir in the milk over a gentle heat. Don't be alarmed that the mixture looks lumpy at this stage.
3 Turn off the heat and quickly stir in the orange juice, egg yolk and chocolate pieces, stirring briskly until the chocolate has melted.
4 Beat the egg white until it forms fairly stiff peaks. Using a metal spoon to prevent air escaping from the beaten egg, take one spoonful and fold gently into the chocolate mixture. Gradually fold the rest of the egg white into the mixture, taking care not to lose the air.
5 Carefully spoon the mixture into individual ramekins and bake for around 25 minutes. If you need to insert a skewer into one of the puddings to check if it's done, you can disguise the damage with some artfully shaken cocoa powder on the top.

PER SERVING: 6

COOK'S NOTES
ALLERGY SUITABILITY gluten, wheat free (check that the chocolate is dairy free if necessary)

PER SERVING: 6

COOK'S NOTES

VARIATIONS use apricots instead
of plums
ALLERGY SUITABILITY gluten, wheat,
dairy, yeast free

Amaretti stuffed plums

Almonds are an excellent source of calcium and protein to keep
the GL score low. Here, plums are lightly baked with a chewy,
almondy biscuit topping – delicious and very healthy.

SERVES 2

100g (4oz) ground almonds
3–4 drops of almond extract
4 organic, free range egg yolks
75g (3oz) xylitol
4 ripe plums, halved and destoned
1 tbsp flaked almonds

1 Preheat the oven to 180C/350F/Gas mark 4, and line
a baking tray with baking paper.
2 Mix together the ground almonds, almond extract,
egg yolks and xylitol to form a thick paste.
3 Shape into 4 balls and press into the middle of each plum
half, then sprinkle with flaked almonds.
4 Place on the baking tray and bake for around 12 minutes
until the top starts to turn golden and the fruit is soft when
squeezed. Don't overcook it or the plums will collapse.

PER SERVING: 7

COOK'S NOTES

ALLERGY SUITABILITY gluten, wheat,
dairy, yeast free

Baked apple with almond custard

Baked apples are a simple pudding and wonderfully warming when
served with this smooth, creamy (but dairy-free) almond custard.

SERVES 2

1 Bramley (cooking) apple, cored then cut
   in half horizontally, unpeeled
1 tbsp flaked almonds

FOR THE ALMOND CUSTARD

1 level tbsp cornflour
210ml (7fl. oz) water
1 heaped tbsp ground almonds
1 heaped tbsp xylitol

1 Preheat the oven to 180C/350F/Gas mark 4.
2 Place the apple halves on a baking tray. Bake for 20 minutes
until soft in the middle but not collapsing.
3 Meanwhile, dry-fry the flaked almonds in a pan until they're
a light golden colour. Set to one side.
4 To make the custard, mix the cornflour with two tablespoons
of the water until smooth. Pour it into a pan with the ground
almonds and xylitol and heat gently, stirring for around 5 minutes
and gradually adding the rest of the water to form a smooth,
thick sauce.
5 Place an apple half on each plate and top with the custard,
then sprinkle the toasted almond flakes on top and serve.

Hazelnut yoghurt

The perfect pudding for when you are in a rush. Full of protein and minerals, it also contains probiotic bacteria from the live yoghurt, which aids digestion. You can double this recipe and store in the fridge for up to 3 days.

SERVES 2
125g (just under 5oz) live natural yoghurt
1 tbsp xylitol
50g (2oz) hazelnuts, finely ground (Tip: a coffee grinder works brilliantly, but clean it thoroughly first!)

Stir all the ingredients together well.

PER SERVING: 2

COOK'S NOTES
SERVING SUGGESTION (PER PERSON) serve over Fruit salad (page 69) (total = 9)
ALLERGY SUITABILITY gluten, wheat free

Tahini yoghurt

Tahini's rich taste and smooth texture make it perfect for puddings – as halvah and other Middle Eastern sweets attest. Here we've sweetened it in this fast, tasty pudding full of omega-6 oils and probiotic bacteria. You can double this recipe and store in the fridge for up to 3 days.

SERVES 2
200g (7oz) live natural yoghurt
4 tbsp tahini
2 tbsp xylitol

Stir all the ingredients well together.

PER SERVING: 4

COOK'S NOTES
ALLERGY SUITABILITY gluten, wheat free

Rhubarb fool

This is a gorgeous pink colour and has all the taste of a classic fruit fool but less fat, as it uses natural yoghurt instead of cream. Serve chilled. You can store it in the fridge for up to 3 days.

SERVES 2
300g (11oz) trimmed rhubarb, washed and cut into chunks
Dash of water
3 tbsp xylitol
200g (7oz) live natural yoghurt

1 Place the rhubarb in a saucepan with the water and xylitol. Simmer for around 10 minutes, uncovered, until soft and disintegrating.
2 Allow the rhubarb to cool, then stir into the yoghurt to create a smooth, pink fool.
3 Spoon into 2 glasses or ramekins and chill until required.

PER SERVING: 6

COOK'S NOTES
VARIATIONS use plums instead of rhubarb – they will need less cooking time
ALLERGY SUITABILITY gluten, wheat free

COOK'S NOTES

VARIATIONS vary the nuts and seeds
in the base if you like
ALLERGY SUITABILITY wheat free

Lemon cheesecake

No, it isn't too good to be true! This delicious treat – perfect for
dinner parties or a tea-time snack – has a biscuit base made from
rough oat cakes, nuts and seeds, and a fabulously rich, lemony
filling. It's wheat-free, low-GL and fibre-rich, and contains plenty
of minerals and essential fats from the nuts and seeds. You can
store this cheesecake covered in the fridge for up to 3 days.

SERVES 8
FOR THE BASE
25g (1oz) coconut oil or butter
15g (just over 1/2 oz) xylitol
50g (2oz) ground almonds
25g (1oz) finely chopped hazelnuts
25g (1oz) finely chopped sunflower seeds and pumpkin seeds
25g (1oz) Nairn's rough, organic oat cakes, ground in a blender
   or food processor
2 tsp ground ginger

FOR THE FILLING
4 medium eggs
5 tbsp xylitol
275g (10oz) low-fat cream cheese
125g (just under 5oz) natural yoghurt
Finely grated zest of 8 lemons (preferably unwaxed)
Juice of 2 lemons
1/2 tsp vanilla extract
4 tbsp cornflour

1 Preheat the oven to 150C/300F/Gas mark 2 and line a medium-
sized tart or cake tin (approximately 23cm/8 1/2in diameter) with
a removable bottom. (Clip-type tins are best as they will not leak.)
2 Very gently melt the oil or butter in a pan (don't let it bubble) and
stir in the xylitol to melt, again taking care not to boil.
3 Remove from the heat and stir in the rest of the base ingredients.
4 Using the underside of a tablespoon, press this mixture firmly into
the bottom of the cake tin to cover it evenly. Bake for 10 minutes,
then set to one side. Do not attempt to dislodge the base at this
 point as it will crumble.
5 Increase the oven temperature to 170C/325F/Gas mark 3.
6 Blend all of the filling ingredients together until smooth.
7 Carefully pour the filling onto the prepared base and place in
a roasting tin to catch any drips from the bottom of the tin.
8 When the oven is up to temperature, bake for 40 to 45 minutes
or until the filling is set. Allow to cool before you cut the cheesecake.

Apricot crunch

If you like nutty chewy granola and flapjacks, you'll love this low-carb, high-protein pudding. Its sweet, nutty crunch topping complements the apricot compote and yoghurt wonderfully, and it can be thrown together in minutes.

PER SERVING: 5

COOK'S NOTES
ALLERGY SUITABILITY gluten, wheat free

SERVES 2
50g (2oz) hazelnuts, finely chopped or ground
4 tsp xylitol
4 apricots, destoned and chopped
Dash of water
200g (7oz) live natural yoghurt

1 Place the hazelnuts and the 4 teaspoons of xylitol in a pan and stir over a gentle heat for a couple of minutes to mix together. Allow to cool.
2 Place the apricots, the remaining 2 teaspoons of xylitol and the water in a separate pan and gently simmer for a couple of minutes, covered, to soften the fruit and produce a compote.
3 Spoon the compote in the bottom of 2 short glasses or 2 large ramekins and pour the yoghurt on top (glasses work best because you can see the different layers of the pudding).
4 Sprinkle the sweetened nuts on top and place in the fridge until ready to serve.

Pear crumble

Crumbles represent the very best of traditional British cooking – simple, but utterly scrumptious. This version uses protein-rich nuts and seeds in the wheatless topping to lower the carb content and GL score. It is also made on the hob, so it's much quicker to cook, and preserves more nutrients. You can double this recipe and store in the fridge for up to 2 days.

SERVES 2
FOR THE PEAR FILLING
2 ripe pears, cored and diced
1/4 tsp ground ginger or 1/2 tsp ground cinnamon
1 tsp lemon juice
1 tsp xylitol

FOR THE CRUMBLE
1 tbsp coconut oil or olive oil
1 tbsp xylitol
50g (2oz) whole oat flakes
1 tbsp flaked almonds
1 tbsp macadamia nuts, roughly chopped
1 tbsp pumpkin seeds
1 tbsp ground almonds

1 For the pear filling, place the pears in a saucepan along with the ginger or cinnamon, lemon juice and the teaspoon of xylitol. Cover and stew gently until the fruit softens, stirring from time to time to prevent it from sticking.
2 While that is cooking, make the crumble. Gently heat the oil in a frying pan with the xylitol, add the oats and fry for 3 minutes, or until they start to colour and harden slightly.
3 Add the flaked almonds and macadamia nuts and cook for a further 2 minutes.
4 Remove from the heat and stir in the pumpkin seeds and ground almonds.
5 Divide the cooked pear between two ramekins and cover with the crumble. Serve warm.

Pear and baked custard pudding

This combination of light baked custard and soft pears has plenty of protein from the egg and yoghurt, and is real nursery food.

SERVES 2
2 medium eggs
2 tbsp xylitol
125g (just under 5oz) live natural yoghurt
1/2 tsp vanilla extract
1 tbsp cornflour
1/2 a ripe pear, cored and thinly sliced

1 Preheat the oven to 170C/325F/Gas mark 3.
2 Whisk the eggs with the xylitol, yoghurt, vanilla extract and cornflour until it forms a smooth liquid.
3 Place the pear slices in the base of a small ovenproof dish and pour the custard mixture on top. Bake for 30 to 35 minutes or until the custard is set and pale golden.

PER SERVING: 4

COOK'S NOTES
VARIATIONS replace the pear with apple or berries
ALLERGY SUITABILITY gluten, wheat free

Almond custard

A dairy-free alternative to traditional custard, and just as smooth and delicious. The wonderful almond flavour works well with stewed or baked fruit.

SERVES 2
1 level tbsp cornflour
210ml (7fl. oz) water
1 heaped tbsp ground almonds
1 heaped tbsp xylitol

1 Mix the cornflour with 2 tablespoons of the water until smooth.
2 Pour it into a pan with the ground almonds and xylitol and heat gently, stirring constantly for around 5 minutes, gradually adding the rest of the water to form a smooth, thick sauce.

PER SERVING: 2

COOK'S NOTES
ALLERGY SUITABILITY gluten, wheat, dairy, yeast free

MAINTENANCE PHASE
serve over the fruit compotes (page 69) (total = 7) or with Pear crumble (see page 168) (total = 9)

Rice pudding

Chopped nuts add an unusual and delicious twist to our version of the carb-rich comfort food. Brown basmati rice has the lowest GL score of all types of rice, while yoghurt increases the protein content and provides a creamy consistency.

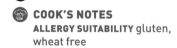

PER SERVING: 6

COOK'S NOTES
ALLERGY SUITABILITY gluten, wheat free

SERVES 2
100g (4oz) brown basmati rice
210ml (7fl oz) water
100g (4oz) natural yoghurt
4 tsp xylitol
2 tsp lemon juice
1 tbsp chopped, unsalted and unroasted nuts (such as shelled pistachios, walnuts, pecans, Brazil nuts or almonds)

1 Put the rice and water in a small saucepan and bring to the boil, then cover and simmer for 15 minutes until the rice is al dente and the water has been absorbed.
2 Add the yoghurt, xylitol and lemon juice, stir and gently heat to melt the yoghurt and form a sauce. Don't let the yoghurt boil or it will separate.
3 Spoon into 2 ramekins and sprinkle the chopped nuts on top.

Banana and berry frozen yoghurt

Ice cream is fairly low GL, but high in fat and sugar. This is a brilliant alternative. It gets its sweetness from fruit and its creaminess from mashed banana and yoghurt. Absolutely fabulous!

PER SERVING: 6

COOK'S NOTES
ALLERGY SUITABILITY gluten, wheat free

SERVES 2
1 small banana
300g (11oz) live natural yoghurt
4 heaped tbsp mixed berries, such as strawberries, raspberries, blackberries or blueberries (fresh, or frozen and defrosted)

1 Mash the banana and place in a bowl with the yoghurt and berries, stirring them together.
2 Tip into a plastic container, seal with a lid and place in the freezer for 2 hours to chill and harden. Mash up with a fork before serving to soften any ice crystals that have formed. If you leave it in the freezer for longer before serving, you should let it sit at room temperature for a while to soften before you try to mash it, as otherwise it will be very hard and icy.

LOW-GL PANCAKES

These pancakes are just as delicious as the ones we stuffed ourselves with on Shrove Tuesday when we were small. We've simply used high-protein in order to lower the GL score. It also means the pancakes are gluten free.

Blueberry pancakes

Delicious blueberry compote oozing out of sweet pancakes – yum. Blueberries are a superfood, rich in powerful antioxidants.

MAKES 4 LARGE PANCAKES (TO SERVE 4 OR 2 – SEE BELOW)

FOR THE PANCAKES

50g (2oz) cornflour
50g (2oz) quinoa flour
35g (around 1 1/2 oz) xylitol
210ml (7fl.oz) skimmed milk, soya milk or nut milk
2 1/2 tbsp water
1 medium egg
4 tsp coconut oil for frying (1 tsp per pancake)

FOR THE FILLING

4 tbsp blueberries
2 tsp xylitol
1 tbsp water
1 tsp lemon juice

1 Make the pancakes by blending all the pancake ingredients except the coconut oil in a blender until smooth.
2 Melt one teaspoon of the coconut oil in a frying pan and tip to coat the whole pan surface. Spoon in half a ladleful of the batter (a quarter of the total batter) and tip the pan to spread it evenly in a circle around the base.
3 Cook for 30 to 45 seconds, then turn with a spatula (or the more adventurous can attempt to flip) and cook the other side for a similar length of time, until pale golden.
4 Remove from the pan and keep warm (place on a plate and cover with a clean, dry tea towel) until it is ready to be served. You will have to add another teaspoon of oil to the pan between pancakes to make sure they do not stick.
5 To make the blueberry filling, place the blueberries in a pan with the xylitol, water and lemon juice and heat gently until the berries starts to burst and release their juice, producing a berry compote. Spoon a bit into the middle of each pancake and fold up.

(GL) PER SERVING: 4 PER PANCAKE

COOK'S NOTES
SERVING SUGGESTION (PER PERSON)
have 1 pancake
VARIATIONS for other fillings, squeeze fresh lemon juice over the pancake and sprinkle with xylitol, then roll up; fill with Fruit compote (see page 69) and crème fraîche; or sprinkle grated dark chocolate and chopped pistachios over, then roll up
ALLERGY SUITABILITY gluten, wheat, dairy, yeast free

MAINTENANCE PHASE
have 2 pancakes (total (GL) = 8)

Almond pancakes

Almonds are rich in calcium and magnesium, and make a deliciously crunchy filling for almond-flavoured pancakes.

MAKES 4 LARGE PANCAKES (TO SERVE 4 OR 2 – SEE BELOW)
FOR THE PANCAKES
50g (2oz) cornflour
50g (2oz) quinoa flour
35g (around 1$\frac{1}{2}$ oz) xylitol
210ml (7fl. oz) skimmed milk, soya milk or nut milk
$\frac{1}{2}$ tsp almond extract
2 $\frac{1}{2}$ tbsp water
1 medium egg
4 tsp coconut oil for frying (1 tsp per pancake)

FOR THE FILLING
4 heaped tbsp flaked almonds
4 tbsp lemon juice
1 tbsp xylitol

1 Blend all of the pancake ingredients except the coconut oil in a blender until smooth.
2 Melt one teaspoon of the coconut oil in a frying pan and tip to coat the whole pan surface. Spoon in half a ladleful of the batter (a quarter of the total batter) and tip the pan to spread it evenly in a circle around the base.
3 Cook for 30 to 45 seconds, then turn with a spatula (or the more adventurous can attempt to flip) and cook the other side for a similar length of time, until pale golden.
4 Remove from the pan and keep warm (place on a plate and cover with a clean, dry tea towel) until it is to be served. You will have to add another teaspoon of coconut oil to the pan between pancakes to make sure they do not stick.
5 To make the filling, keep the pan on a low heat after making the pancakes and place the flaked almonds in the pan. As soon as the nuts start to turn golden add the xylitol and lemon juice – the mixture will sizzle and form a sweet sauce.
6 Immediately spoon the nut sauce into the middle of each pancake and roll up.

Cheese platter

If you like rounding off a meal with cheese and biscuits, try our low-GL version – which also boosts your vitamin and essential fats intake via veg or fruit and nuts.

SERVES 2
4 Nairn's rough oat cakes
either 100g (4oz) cubed feta or goat's cheese
or 200g (7oz) low-fat cottage cheese

WITH EITHER
1 carrot, cut into batons and
1 stick of celery, cut into batons
OR
1 tart apple (such as Braeburn), sliced and
1 handful of walnut halves, pecans or Brazil nuts

Arrange the ingredients on a platter and serve.

PER SERVING: 6

COOK'S NOTES
VARIATIONS use cucumber instead of celery, and pear instead of apple
ALLERGY SUITABILITY wheat free

Almond shortbread

Rich and wonderfully crumbly, shortbread is the sort of thing we all crave when cutting down on carbs. Our version uses low-GL quinoa flour to raise the protein level and makes ample use of ground nuts. The result is even crumblier than the traditional version, and just as mouthwatering. These will keep in an airtight tin for up to 3 days.

SERVES 2
25g (1oz) coconut oil or butter, at room temperature (if the coconut oil is still hard, heat it very slightly to get it to the same consistency as softened butter)
25g (1oz) xylitol
25g (1oz) ground almonds
50g (2oz) quinoa flour
1 handful of flaked almonds

1 Preheat the oven to 170C/325F/Gas mark 3 and line a small baking tray with nonstick paper.
2 Beat the coconut oil or butter and xylitol using an electric whisk until light and creamy.
3 Rub the ground almonds and quinoa flour into the mixture using your fingertips, working lightly – the mixture should soon resemble breadcrumbs.
4 Press the mixture evenly into the lined baking tin to form a square about 1/2 in thick (don't worry that it doesn't cover the entire tray), sprinkle with flaked almonds and bake for 20 minutes.
5 Allow to cool on a wire rack, then cut into 4 squares and store in an airtight container.

PER SERVING: 4

COOK'S NOTES
SERVING SUGGESTION (PER PERSON) have 2 each
VARIATIONS use hazelnuts in place of almonds
ALLERGY SUITABILITY gluten, wheat, dairy, yeast free

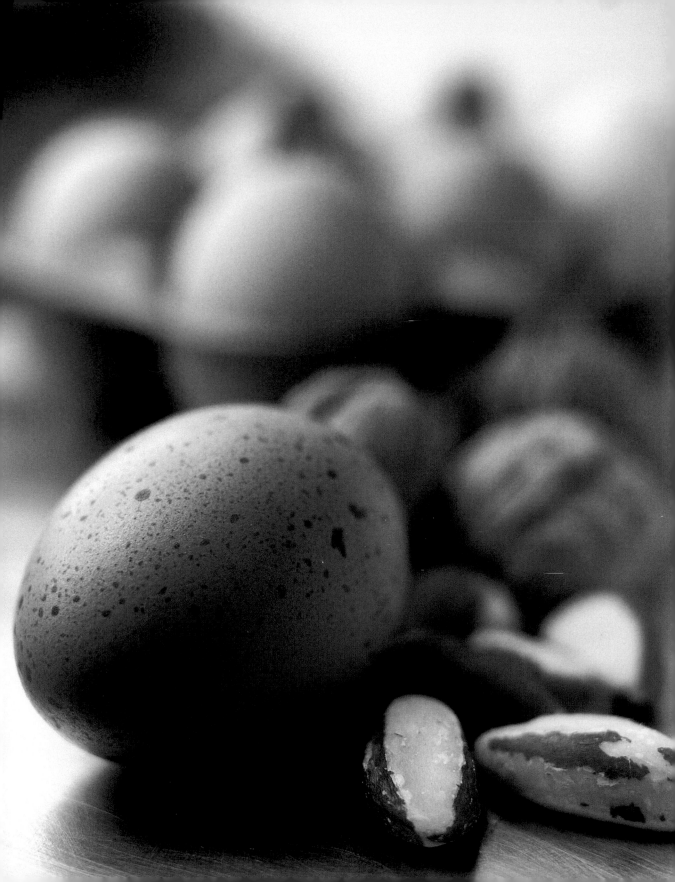

Apricot amaretti biscuits

We use this recipe at cookery demonstrations, as it's the perfect example of how quick, easy and tasty optimum nutrition cooking can be. It is gluten, dairy, yeast and sugar free with no added fat, yet high in fibre and essential fats, low-GL – and utterly delicious. These will keep in an airtight tin for up to 2 days or you can freeze any that you don't eat straight away.

MAKES 20 SLICES (1 SLICE PER SERVING)

300g (11oz) ground almonds
200g (7oz) xylitol
100g (4oz) cornflour
1 tsp almond extract (not artificial almond flavour), or to taste
4 eggs
1 x 290 tin of apricot halves in unsweetened fruit juice, drained
  (or fresh apricots when in season)
3 good handfuls of flaked almonds

1 Preheat the oven to 180C/350F/Gas mark 4. Line a medium-sized baking tray (23 x 32cm/9 x 12in) with non-stick paper.
2 Combine the ground almonds, xylitol, cornflour, almond extract and eggs and mix thoroughly until smooth. Spoon onto the lined baking tray and smooth out.
3 Lightly press the apricot halves evenly into the base, then sprinkle the flaked almonds on top.
4 Bake for around 20 to 25 minutes, until the top is light golden (check after 20 minutes). Cut into 20 slices.

PER SERVING: 3

COOK'S NOTES
SERVING SUGGESTIONS (PER PERSON) have 1 slice
VARIATIONS omit the apricots
ALLERGY SUITABILITY gluten, wheat, dairy, yeast free

LOW-GL CAKES

Yes, you can have your cake and eat it! These wonderful cake recipes can be served as puddings, or as healthy snacks, and neither of them compromises on taste or texture.

Note: These cakes are baked in a miniature cake tin, available from kitchen shops. If you want to bake a full-sized cake (serving 16), multiply the quantities given by 4, use a standard cake tin (approximately 23cm/ 8½in diameter) and increase the cooking time. As this is a dense cake it may take around 1½–2 hours to cook, depending on your oven. Cover with foil after 45 minutes to an hour to stop the top from burning, and check if it is cooked every so often by inserting a skewer in the middle – it should come out coated in crumbs rather than with gloopy raw cake mixture.

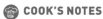

⊕ PER SERVING: 5

👩‍🍳 COOK'S NOTES

VARIATIONS replace the apple with pears. You could also use quinoa flour instead of soya flour, although the flavour is not as good
ALLERGY SUITABILITY gluten, wheat, dairy, yeast free (use coconut oil rather than butter if you cannot eat dairy)

Apple and almond cake

This recipe is a healthier version of Fiona's all-time favourite, Dorset apple cake, which is overflowing with butter and sugar. You'll get all the taste and texture of the original here, but without the gluten, sugar and dairy, plus fibre and minerals instead. The soya flour also provides phytoestrogens for hormone balance. This cake will keep in an airtight tin for up to 2 days.

SERVES 4
50g (2oz) coconut oil or butter (at room temperature)
50g (2oz) xylitol
50g (2oz) organic soya flour (available from health food stores)
½ tsp baking powder
50g (2oz) ground almonds
50g (2oz) flaked almonds plus 1 tbsp for sprinkling on top
150g (5oz) Bramley (cooking) apples (cored weight), unpeeled and diced
2 medium eggs

1 Preheat the oven to 180C/350F/Gas mark 4. Grease and line a miniature 10cm/4in cake tin with non-stick paper. Alternatively, you could use 2 medium-sized muffin moulds, lined with paper liners.
2 Cream the coconut oil or butter and xylitol together until soft and smooth.
3 Stir in the flour, baking powder and ground almonds until the mixture resembles breadcrumbs.
4 Mix in the flaked almonds (reserving 1 tbsp) and apples, then stir in the eggs without beating them.
5 Spoon into the prepared cake tin and sprinkle the reserved flaked almonds on top. Bake for 25 minutes or until the top is golden and set. Remove from the oven and cover the top with a sheet of tin foil, then return to the oven for a further 20 minutes or until the cake is cooked. (Tip: insert a skewer into the middle – if it comes out fairly clean then the cake is cooked; if it is still runny then it needs a bit longer.)

Carrot and walnut cake

Another fabulous tea-time treat that you can enjoy without feeling guilty. The walnuts, carrots and eggs in this cake lower the GL score and provide plenty of varied nutrients. Delicious with a cup of peppermint tea at the end of a long day. If you use the walnut topping, this cake will keep in an airtight tin for up to 2 days. If you opt for the cream cheese frosting, cover the cake and store in the fridge for 2 days.

SERVES 4
FOR THE CAKE
50g (2oz) coconut oil or butter (at room temperature)
50g (2oz) xylitol
50g (2oz) organic soya flour (available from health food stores)
¼ tsp baking powder
50g (2oz) ground walnuts
50g (2oz) chopped walnuts
1 medium carrot (approximately 75g/3oz) peeled and finely grated
2 medium eggs

FOR THE TOPPING
EITHER
CREAM CHEESE FROSTING
50g (2oz) low fat cream cheese
½ tsp vanilla extract
1 tsp xylitol

OR
WALNUT TOPPING
2 tbsp chopped walnuts

1 Preheat the oven to 180C/350F/Gas mark 4. Grease and line a miniature 10cm/4in cake tin with non-stick paper.
2 Cream the coconut oil or butter and xylitol together until soft and smooth.
3 Stir in the flour, baking powder and ground walnuts until the mixture resembles breadcrumbs.
4 Mix in the chopped walnuts and carrot, then stir in the eggs without beating them.
5 Spoon into the prepared cake tin and sprinkle the chopped walnuts on top, if using. Bake for 35 minutes or until the top is risen and golden. Remove from the oven and cover the top with tin foil, then bake for a further 20 minutes or until the cake is cooked. (Tip: insert a skewer into the middle – if it comes out fairly clean then the cake is cooked, if it is still runny then it needs a bit longer). Allow to cool before icing with the cream cheese frosting, if using.
6 To make the cream cheese frosting, mix all the frosting ingredients together well. Spread on top of the cooled cake.

PER SERVING: 5

COOK'S NOTES
VARIATIONS you could also use quinoa flour (another high protein flour, from health food stores) instead of soya flour, although the flavour is not as good
ALLERGY SUITABILITY gluten, wheat, dairy, yeast free (opt for the chopped walnut topping rather than the frosting if you cannot eat dairy products or yeast, and use coconut oil rather than butter if you cannot eat dairy)

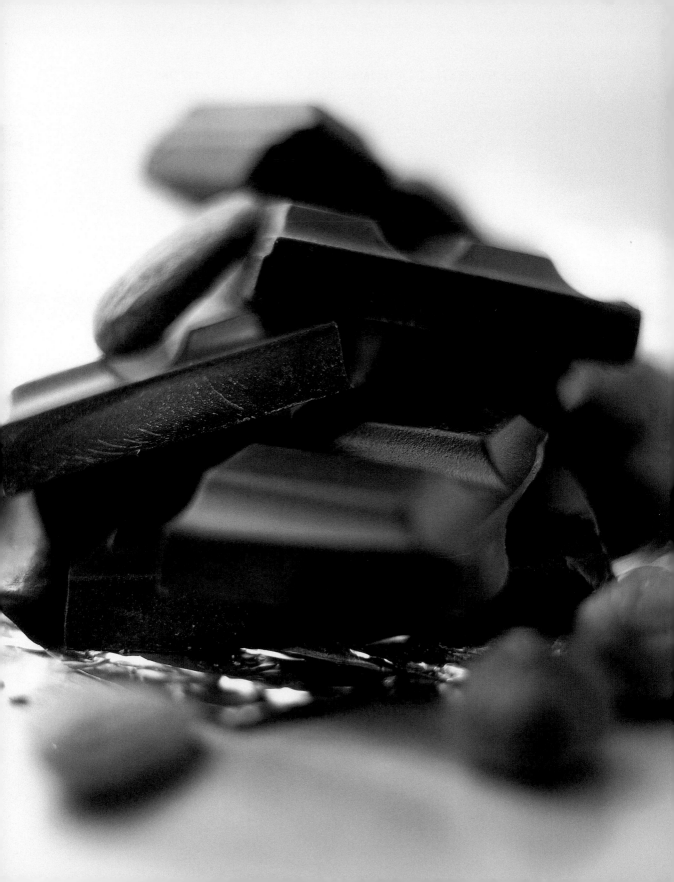

Marzipan truffles

These luscious, almondy truffles wouldn't be out of place served at a dinner party or smartly packaged and given as presents (note, though, that they must stay chilled). Marzipan lends itself well to low-GL sweets, as the nuts and eggs provide protein with minimal carbohydrate. These will keep chilled in the fridge for up to 24 hours.

MAKES 8 TRUFFLES (4 PER SERVING)
125g (just under 5oz) ground almonds
4 drops almond extract
75g (3oz) xylitol
4 organic, free range egg yolks
1 heaped tbsp finely chopped almonds

1 Mix the ground almonds, almond extract, xylitol and egg yolks together until they form a smooth paste.
2 Shape into walnut-sized balls and roll each ball in a saucer of the finely chopped almonds until the outside is coated in nuts.
3 Place on a plate and store in the fridge till firm.

PER SERVING: 5

COOK'S NOTES
SERVING SUGGESTION (PER PERSON)
serve 4 per person
ALLERGY SUITABILITY gluten, wheat, dairy, yeast free

> **HEALTH NOTE: BECAUSE THIS RECIPE CONTAINS RAW EGG, ALWAYS CHOOSE ORGANIC OR AT THE VERY LEAST FREE RANGE EGGS TO REDUCE THE LIKELIHOOD OF SALMONELLA CONTAMINATION, AND DO NOT SERVE TO PREGNANT WOMEN, YOUNG CHILDREN, THE ELDERLY OR INFIRM.**

Chocolate dipped nuts

A sweet treat that is positively good for you – the nuts are high in protein and minerals, and dark chocolate is low in sugar and rich in magnesium. You can double this recipe and store the remainder in the fridge for up to 10 days.

SERVES 2 (4 PER SERVING)
15g (around ½ oz) good quality dark chocolate, broken into pieces
25g (1oz) shelled mixed nuts (such as almonds, macadamia nuts, hazelnuts, Brazil nuts or cashews)

1 Line a baking tray with non-stick paper.
2 Gently melt the chocolate. To do this, half fill a saucepan with water and let simmer. Place the chocolate in a small metal or heat-proof bowl that fits the rim of the saucepan but does not touch the water, and allow it to melt over the heat, stirring occasionally.
3 Tip the nuts into the melted chocolate and stir to coat. Place the nuts on the baking tray, making sure they are not touching – otherwise they will stick together when they harden.
4 When all the nuts are done, place the tray in the fridge to let the chocolate harden completely.

PER SERVING: 4

COOK'S NOTES
SERVING SUGGESTION (PER PERSON)
serve a small handful each
ALLERGY SUITABILITY gluten, wheat, dairy, yeast free (make sure you choose dairy-free chocolate if necessary)

DRINKS

While water, herbal teas and a daily glass of diluted juice are the drinks we recommend on Holford Diet, there are moments – particularly at parties, or snacktime on a hot summer day – when you yearn for something a bit different. So in addition to the 5 ⒼⓁ drinks listed in Part 1 on page 33, we have included some scrummy recipes that will inspire you to abandon fizzy drinks and squashes once and for all.

Caffe lattes don't have a place in this section, either. As you'll now probably know, caffeinated drinks mess up your blood sugar control, with knock-on effects on your weight and energy. Alcohol, too, is problematic in this context, but remember that you can have the occasional glass of wine (see page 33) and, for special occasions and parties, we've even included a couple of delicious cocktails in this section – see Cook's Notes for the Gingerade and Lemonade recipes below.

Remember: Your drinks and/or pudding allowance is 5 ⒼⓁ in total for weight loss and 10 ⒼⓁ for maintenance.

RECIPE	ⒼⓁ SCORE
Apple, lemon and ginger smoothie **p.182**	5
Pear and blueberry smoothie **p.182**	4
St Clement's smoothie **p.182**	3
Strawberry smoothie **p.183**	3
Gingerade **p.183**	1
Lemonade **p.184**	1
Virgin Mary **p.184**	4

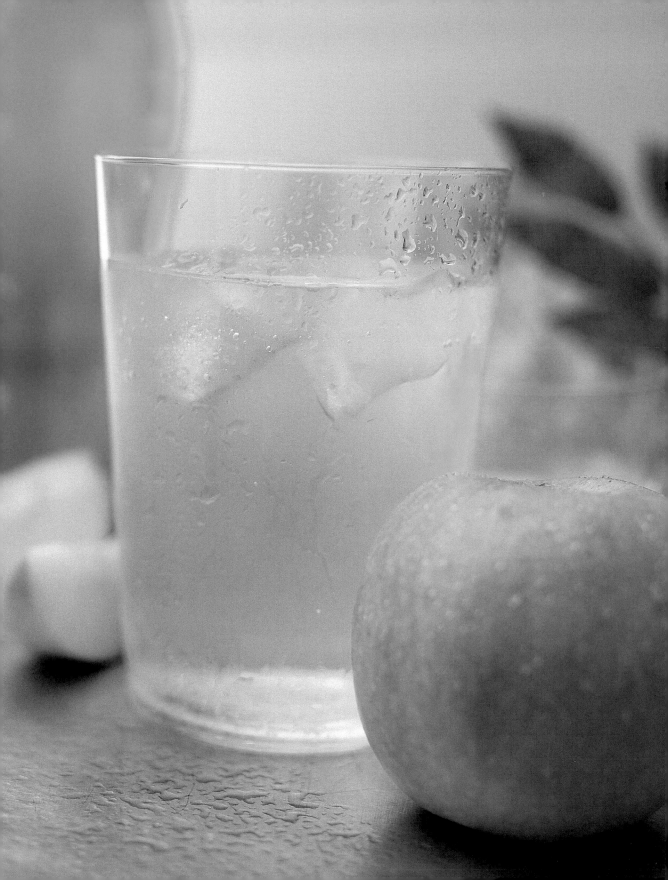

Apple, lemon and ginger smoothie

 PER SERVING: 5

COOK'S NOTES
VARIATIONS omit the ginger if preferred
ALLERGY SUITABILITY gluten, wheat, dairy free

This soothing apple smoothie with a ginger and citrus kick provides a real vitamin C boost. Leave the apple peel on for more nutrients – it blends down quite well.

SERVES 2
2 small apples, cored and diced
200g (7oz) live natural yoghurt or soya yoghurt
2 tsp lemon juice
Good pinch of dried ginger

1 Blend the ingredients together, using a handheld blender, until smooth.
2 Chill if you like, then pour into 2 glasses and serve.

Pear and blueberry smoothie

 PER SERVING: 4

COOK'S NOTES
VARIATIONS use an apple instead of the pear. Use the same quantity of skimmed milk, or soya milk or nut milk in place of yoghurt for a thinner, shake-style drink
ALLERGY SUITABILITY gluten, wheat free

A thick and yummy superfood smoothie with juicy, antioxidant-packed blueberries and pear for natural sweetness.

SERVES 2
1 pear
2 tbsp blueberries
200g (7oz) live natural yoghurt

1 Blend the ingredients together, using a handheld blender, until smooth.
2 Chill if you like, then pour into 2 glasses and serve.

St Clement's smoothie

PER SERVING: 3

COOK'S NOTES
ALLERGY SUITABILITY gluten, wheat free

Creamy yoghurt and sweet oranges, with a distinct lemony tang – this vitamin C-rich drink is very refreshing.

SERVES 2
Juice of two oranges
Juice of one lemon
200g (7oz) live natural yoghurt

1 Blend the ingredients together, using a handheld blender, until smooth.
2 Chill if you like, then pour into 2 short glasses and serve.

Strawberry smoothie

This refreshing summer smoothie is bursting with phytonutrients from the vivid red pigment in the strawberries.

SERVES 2

450g (1lb) stawberries, rinsed and drained then hulled
200g (7oz) live natural yoghurt or soya yoghurt

1 Blend the ingredients together, using a handheld blender, until smooth.
2 Chill if you like, then pour into 2 short glasses and serve.

PER SERVING: 3

COOK'S NOTES
VARIATIONS use different berries, such as raspberries or blackberries, or a mixture
ALLERGY SUITABILITY gluten, wheat, dairy free

Gingerade

A wonderful sugar free version of gingerade. It's a good idea to include ginger in your diet regularly: not only does fresh ginger add bags of flavour to both sweet and savoury meals, it is also a powerful immune booster with antiviral and antibacterial properties.

SERVES 2

1 heaped tbsp xylitol
50g (2oz) chunk of fresh root ginger, peeled and cut into large chunks (Tip: the easiest way to peel fresh ginger is by scraping the skin off with the edge of a teaspoon)
300ml (1/2 pt) still water
300ml (1/2 pt) chilled sparking mineral water

1 Place the xylitol, root ginger and still water in a pan and bring to the boil.
2 Cover and simmer for around 10 minutes, then remove from the heat and leave to cool before removing the ginger pieces.
3 Stir the syrup liquid into the sparkling mineral water and serve.

PER SERVING: 1

COOK'S NOTES
SERVING SUGGESTION (PER PERSON) serve with ice cubes and a slice of lemon
VARIATIONS add 1 shot of vodka per person to turn this into a fabulous Moscow Mule for summer evenings
ALLERGY SUITABILITY gluten, wheat, dairy, yeast free

Lemonade

Homemade lemonade is the essence of summer – super-refreshing and chockfull of vitamin C. In our version, xylitol provides all the sweetness but fewer calories and carbs than sugar.

SERVES 2
juice of 4 lemons
1 tbsp xylitol
600ml (1pt) chilled sparkling mineral water

1 Place the lemon juice and xylitol in a pan and gently heat until the xylitol dissolves.
2 Allow to cool, then stir into the sparkling mineral water and serve.

Virgin Mary

After a long day at work, a spicy-hot Virgin Mary is a great way to chill out, and it's packed with vitamins too. (You can quadruple the recipe and keep in the fridge for up to 3 days, so it's ready when you walk through the door.) Or you can order this when out with friends, but avoiding alcohol.

SERVES 2 (IN SHORT GLASSES)
1 x 330ml can V8 (vegetable) juice or tomato juice
1 tsp lemon juice
Freshly ground black pepper
6 drops of hot pepper sauce or Tabasco, or to taste
6 drops of Worcestershire sauce, or to taste (optional)

Mix all the ingredients together and pour into 2 short glasses and serve.

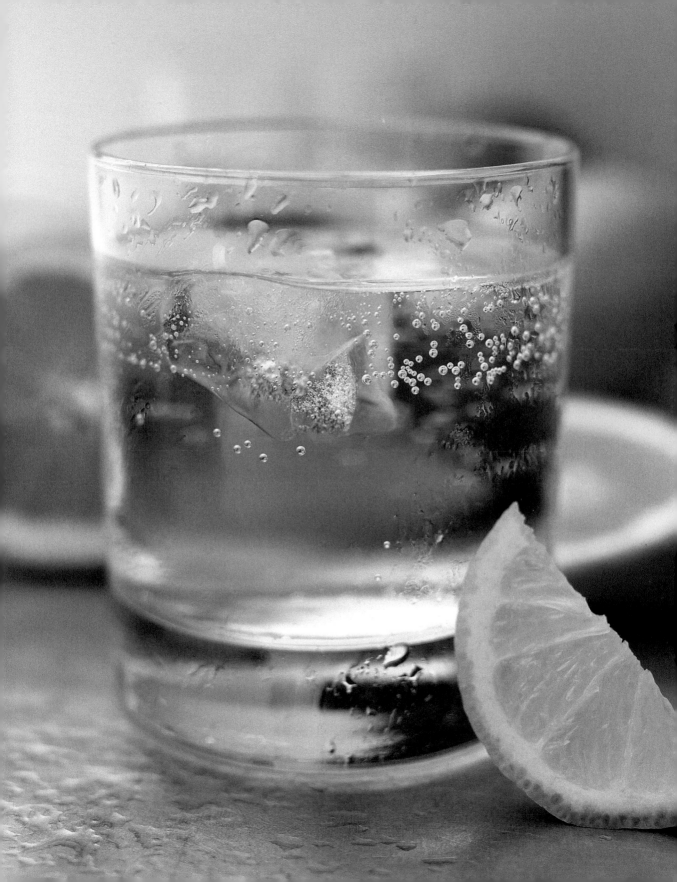

RECOMMENDED READING

Holford, Patrick, *The Optimum Nutrition Bible*, Piatkus (2009).
Holford, Patrick and Judy Ridgway, *The Optimum Nutrition Cookbook*, Piatkus (2010).
Holford, Patrick, *The Low-GL Diet Bible*, Piatkus (2009).

RESOURCES

Cookery Clinics
Fiona McDonald Joyce is a trained nutritionist and cookery consultant to commercial caterers and private individuals. If you would like her help with recipe development, or menu or dietary advice, she can be contacted via fmcdj@hotmail.com.

Institute for Optimum Nutrition (ION)

ION runs the Home Study Course and the three-year Nutrition Therapists' Foundation Degree course. For details on courses, consultations and publications send a stamped, addressed envelope to ION, Ambassador House, Paradise Road, Richmond, Surrey TW9 1SQ. Telephone: +44 (0)20 8614 7800; or fax: +44 (0)870 979 1133.

Nutrition consultations
To find a nutritional therapist in your area visit www.bant.org.uk (the British Association for Applied Nutrition and Nutritional Therapy). If there is no one available nearby, you can always take an online assessment – see below.

Online 100% Health programme
Are you 100 per cent healthy? Find out with our health check and comprehensive, personalised 100% Health Programme giving you an action plan for optimum health, including advice on diet and supplements. Visit www.patrickholford.com.

Psychocalisthenics

Psychocalisthenics is an excellent exercise system that takes less than 20 minutes a day, develops strength, suppleness and stamina, and generates vital energy. The best way to learn it is to do the Psychocalisthenics training courses. Visit www.patrickholford.com (events) for details on these. Also available is the book *Master Level Exercise: Psychocalisthenics*, and the Psychocalisthenics CD and DVD. For further information please see www.pcals.com.

Low-GL foods

Solo Low Sodium Sea Salt
The average person gets far too much sodium because we eat too much salt (sodium chloride) and salted foods, and not enough potassium and magnesium, found in fruits and vegetables. Not all salt, however, is bad for you. Solo Low Sodium Sea Salt contains 60 per cent less sodium and is high in the essential minerals of magnesium and potassium. It is sold in the UK, Ireland, Spain, the Netherlands, Singapore, Hong Kong, Japan, Bahrain, Saudi Arabia, United Arab Emirates, Jordan, the Baltic states and the US. Visit their website www.soloseasalt.com for more information or call: +44 (0)20 8464 1665.

Xylitol

While it is best to avoid sugar and sugar alternatives as much as possible there are two natural sugars that have the lowest GL score. These are blue agave syrup, which is used to sweeten healthier drinks, and xylitol. Xylitol has a GL score a seventh that of regular sugar yet tastes the same. Xylitol is available from Totally Nourish: visit www.totallynourish.com.

Low-GL Get Up and Go

Low-GL Get Up and Go is the perfect Holford Diet breakfast – a delicious, creamy superfood smoothie mix, made from powdered wholefoods, that you blend with strawberries and banana. It's available from good health food stores, or direct from Totally Nourish (call 0800 0857749 or visit www.totallynourish.com).

Tests

Food or chemical allergy and intolerance

YorkTest sell a home test kit for food and chemical allergies that requires a pinprick blood sample. You don't have to go to your doctor. YorkTest laboratories will test you for sensitivity to all foods including gluten, gliadin, wheat and yeast. Visit www.yorktest.com for more information and prices, or call freephone 0800 074 6185 for a Food Sensitivity Test kit.

REFERENCES

[1] K. Heaton et al., 'Particle size of wheat, maize and oat test meals: effects on plasma glucose and insulin responses and on the rate of starch digestion in vitro', *American Journal of Clinical Nutrition*, Vol 47 (1988), pp. 675–82

[2] E. Cheraskin, 'The Breakfast/Lunch/Dinner Ritual', *Journal of Orthomolecular Medicine*, Vol 8(1) (1993), pp. 6–10

[3] J. T. Braaten et al., 'High beta-glucan oat bran and oat gum reduce postprandial blood glucose and insulin in subjects with and without type 2 diabetes', *Diabetic Medicine*, Vol 11(3) (1994), pp. 312–18

[4] C. Ebbeling et al., 'A reduced-glycemic load diet in the treatment of obesity', *Archives of Pediatrics and Adolescent Medicine*, Vol 157 (8) (2003), pp. 773–9

[5] C. M. Albert et al., 'Blood levels of long-chain n-3 fatty acids and the risk of sudden death', *New England Journal of Medicine*, Vol 346(15) (2002), pp. 1113–18

[6] M. Morris et al., *Archives of Neurology*, Vol 60 (2003), pp. 940–6

[7] Garg A., 'High mono-unsaturated fat diets for patients with diabetes mellitus: a meta-analysis', *American Journal of Clinical Nutrition*, Vol 67 (1998) (suppl), pp. 577S–582S

[8] T. Hung et al., 'Fat versus carbohydrate in insulin resistance, obesity, diabetes and cardiovascular disease', *Current Opinion in Clinical Nutrition and Metabolic Care*, Vol 6 (2) (2003), pp. 165–76

INDEX

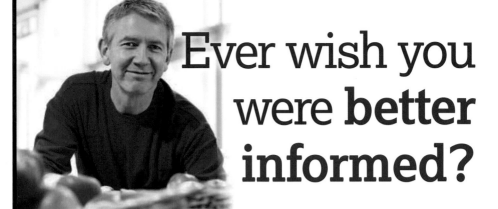

Ever wish you were **better** informed?

Join my 100% Health Club today and you'll receive:

✔ My newsletter, plus Special Reports on vital health topics

✔ Immediate access to hundreds of health articles and special reports.

✔ Have your questions answered in our Members Only blogs.

✔ Save money on supplements, books and other health products.

✔ Save up to £50 on Patrick Holford's **100% Health Workshop**.

✔ Become part of a community of like-minded people and help others.

JOIN TODAY at **www.patrickholford.com**

> ❝ Being a member has transformed my life, and that of many of my family and friends. Patrick's information is always spot on and really practical. My member benefits and discounts save me much more than the subscription. Being a member is a must if you want to be and stay healthy. ❞

Joyce Taylor